Color Atlas of
The Tongue
in Clinical Diagnosis

D.W. Beaven   S.E. Brooks

Color Atlas of
THE
TONGUE
in Clinical Diagnosis

D. W. Beaven

MB ChB (NZ), FRACP, FRCP (Lond), FRCP (Ed), FACP (Hon.)

S. E. Brooks

FNZIMBI FNZIMSI (Hon)

*The Christchurch School of Medicine, University of Otago,
The Princess Margaret Hospital, Christchurch, New Zealand*

With a foreword and assistance with illustrations by **Martin M. Ferguson**, BSc, MB ChB, BDS, FDSRCPS (Glas.) Professor of Oral Medicine and Oral Surgery, University of Otago, Dunedin, New Zealand.

Year Book Medical Publishers, Inc.

To Gwenda and Terry and to Dorothy and June, to whom we owe so much and without whose valuable and dedicated assistance, this book would not have been possible.

Copyright © D.W.Beaven, S.E.Brooks 1988
Published by Wolfe Medical Publications Ltd, 1988
Printed by W.S.Cowell, Ipswich, England

ISBN 0 8151 0587 8
TIF-1

Contents

Foreword

The mouth represents one of the most complex areas of the body with regard to the broad range of disorders affecting it. By virtue of its partial ectodermal and endodermal embryonic origins, the oral mucosa may show manifestations of disease involving skin or gut. In addition, there is a multitude of local problems which are specific to the mouth.

Oral mucosa is extremely sensitive to metabolic disturbances, perhaps only paralleled by the bone marrow, and thus serves as an excellent marker for such disorders. It can be inspected directly and is readily biopsied if necessary.

Unfortunately, diseases of the soft tissue of the mouth tend to fall between the clinical disciplines of medicine and surgery, and medical curricula may omit oral disease entirely. Teaching in dermatology stops at the vermilion border of the lips; ENT discusses the tonsils and pharynx; gastroenterology commences with the oesophagus. Yet when one examines the nature of complaints in patients attending general medical practice, there is a significant number who have symptoms related to the mouth. Medical schools are at last starting to take cognisance of this fact and are incorporating a modicum of teaching about the mouth at undergraduate level. There seems to be a slower move towards including such training in appropriate postgraduate courses.

The publication of this book is most welcome as it focuses on disorders of the tongue, tissue well-recognised as reflecting systemic diseases since the earliest origins of medicine. The ample illustrations provide an excellent review of the range of lesions which can develop, and accordingly should be a valuable guide for those pursuing many training pathways.

Martin M. Ferguson

Acknowledgements

We have been grateful over many years for the interests of colleagues in the teaching hospitals in Christchurch, who have drawn our attention to unusual tongue conditions. Many of these have notified us of their patients and we would like to acknowledge their assistance even when not named on this page.

Mrs Sally Collins, Charge Nurse of the Professorial Medical Unit at The Princess Margaret Hospital, has cast her eye over thousands of acute medical admissions over the last 20 years, drawing our attention to unusual tongues at an early stage in their admission. We are, of course, greatly indebted to her in these and other clinical matters.

Professor Martin Ferguson of the Department of Oral Medicine and Oral Surgery, University of Otago, Dunedin, has given us valuable assistance in lending us many slides, particularly in the area of leukoplakia and lichen planus from his Scottish experience in Oral Medicine. Professor A. C. Smillie of the Department of Oral Biology and Oral Pathology at the University of Otago Medical School, Dunedin, has also given help and loaned slides.

We have greatly valued the cooperation and willing assistance of Dr James Marshall and the staff at Templeton Hospital and Training School, Christchurch, including his dental surgeon, Mrs Mary Livingstone. Dr Marshall's knowledge of each of his in-patients and day-patients, including their background and chromosomal status, was invaluable for the chapter on congenital abnormalities.

Mr Kevin Scally of the Dental Department, Christchurch Hospital, from his close personal association with Dr Ron Every and from his research background, provided us with assistance and understanding.

Mrs Fiona Van Oyen from the Medical Illustrations Department, The Princess Margaret Hospital, and the staff of the Department of Medical Illustrations, both at Christchurch Hospital and The Princess Margaret Hospital, have given great assistance, not only with the production of this book, but also when volunteering as normal subjects. Others who have most kindly contributed slides of patients with unusual tongue conditions and to whom we are very grateful are as follows.

Dr Heather Lyttle from the Sexually Transmitted Diseases Clinic, Christchurch.

Dr Richard Sainsbury, Senior Lecturer in Medicine and Head of Geriatric Services, The Princess Margaret Hospital, Christchurch.

Dr James Neale, Senior Lecturer in Medicine, Wellington Clinical School.

Drs Peter W. Moller, Ivan MacG. Donaldson, Philip J. Parkin, Ross R. Bailey and G. Barrie Tait, all of the Christchurch School of Medicine, Christchurch.

Dr Gordon I. Nicholson, Head of Gastroenterology Department, Auckland Hospital.

Mr Malcolm H. Robertson and Mr Murray H. Greig, Otorhinolaryngology Department, and Dr Christopher H. Atkinson, Oncology Department, Christchurch Hospital.

Professor Derek North of the University of Auckland School of Medicine.

Dr Richard Meech, Infectious Diseases Physician, Hawkes Bay Hospital Board and the New Zealand Advisory Committee on Infectious Diseases.

Mr David Barker and staff of the Department of Dental Surgery, Christchurch Hospital.

Dr Timothy Maling, Clinical Pharmacologist and Senior Lecturer in Medicine, Wellington.

Dr David Scott and Dr Michael Croxson, both of Middlemore Hospital, Auckland.

Dr D. Scollay, Auckland Hospital, Auckland.

Mr Stuart L. Sinclair, Surgeon to the Plastic Surgery Unit, Burwood Hospital, Christchurch.

Mr Ian Stewart, Head of the Ear, Nose and Throat Department, the University of Otago Medical School, Dunedin Hospital, Dunedin.

Dr David Cooper, Head of the Sexually Transmitted Diseases Department, St Vincent's Hospital, Sydney, Australia.

Professors Eric A. Espiner and Richard A. Donald, Endocrine Department, The Princess Margaret Hospital, Christchurch.

Associate Professor George D. Abbott, Paediatrics Department, Christchurch Hospital, Christchurch.

Associate Professor Barry M. Colls, Christchurch School of Medicine.

Dr Keitha Farmer, Paediatrics Services, Auckland Hospital, Auckland.

Dr Ruthven Laing of Auckland.

Dr Deric Bircham, Audio-Visual Department, Dunedin Hospital, Dunedin.

Associate Professor R. D. Gibson, Radiology Department and Head of Academic Radiology, Christchurch, New Zealand, for the fine angiogram of the tongue.

We are greatly indebted to Dr G. R. Kinghorn of the Department of Genito-Urinary Medicine of the Royal Hallamshire Hospital, Glossop Road, Sheffield, England, a world expert in chancroid and herpes, who most generously made available his syphilitic and herpetic slides of the tongue.

We are also greatly indebted to other physicians and colleagues who have been kind enough to lend slides of the tongue from their patients.

For the willing help of all those normal volunteers – medical and dental students and other patients who were prepared to poke out their tongues and have them photographed – we are most grateful and hope that their contribution may assist others to recognise both normal and abnormal tongues. Lastly, our thanks to our own clinical colleagues and the secretarial staff of the Department of Medicine who have been able to tolerate so many crises in the closing stages of putting this book together.

Preface

For over 150 years the tongue has been looked at in the hope of diagnosing health and disease (Froneip, 1828). From the earliest recorded times until quite recently, examining the tongue has been regarded as essential for a health professional to obtain a better understanding of the whole patient. In western civilisation and in Chinese culture (Chen & Hu, 1983), people seeking health care expect their tongue to be routinely examined.

It is the authors' belief that abnormal tongue conditions often pass unnoticed. Even when seen, they are frequently misinterpreted. Thus we may lose a valuable sign relating to the overall health, to any nutritional deficiencies and to the general medical status of the patient. Following examination of the pulse and fingernails, most patients expect their tongue to be looked at by the doctor, nurse or health worker. The host of mainly very common conditions on which we have concentrated in this book may be more easily correlated with disease patterns by these and other groups.

Because of the growing cost of high technology, and the current world-wide swing towards making more use of physical examinations, we believe the visual appearance of the tongue has been greatly under-utilised in the usual quick physical examination.

This book is directed towards *common tongue changes*, and should be of value to medical students, general practitioners, dentists and nurses, as well as many other allied health workers. This volume is *not* a description of oral pathology, nor of diseases of the gingiva or teeth, but concentrates on the appearance of the tongue surface in a wide range of mainly common conditions.

We hope that the study of the visual appearances of the tongue presented here may allow interpretation of the causes and lead to diagnosis or referral. This may go some way towards correcting what appears to be a deficiency in almost all medical textbooks on physical examination or gastroenterology. Most patients expect the tongue to be looked at. Its observation may lead to hypotheses which are then checked by more detailed clinical observations and laboratory measurements. Thus, through curious visual inspection, one leads on to clinical science with the testing of hypotheses by experiments in the clinical laboratory. It is to the ambulant care room or health centre that we must carry the traditions and new methods of 20th century medical science.

In the rush towards modern laboratory examinations, have we perhaps lost an essential part of the clinical skills taught to a previous generation of students? In commenting on examination of the tongue in 1962, Delp and Manning say, 'This time honoured but simple procedure should never be omitted'.

References

Chen Z.L., Hu Q.F. A general survey of studies on tongue examination since the foundation of the People's Republic of China. *J Tradit Chin Med* 1983, **3** (4), 314-332.

Delp M.H., Manning R.T. *Major Physical Diagnosis*, 7th edn. W.B. Saunders, Philadelphia, 1962, pp49&50.

Chapter 1

The Normal Tongue

The tongue develops in the embryo from the primitive foregut and very early invagination from the blastocyst itself. The rich blood supply necessary for the rapid and almost continuous use of tongue muscles, orginally from the primitive branchial arches, has also produced an ability for rapid multiplication and turnover of surface cells (Williams & Warwick, 1980).

In turn, this rich blood supply provides the means whereby the surface of the tongue has evolved with fine filiform and larger fungiform papillae, increasing the surface area for functional use in both taste and mastication.

In the developing infant the tongue is an important sensory organ, exploring a wide variety of ingestible materials. These can be as diverse as sharp or dangerous objects buried in or consumed with primitive foods or tough, indigestible materials. In evolution many ingested nutrients were more hazardous, with most poisons having a bitter taste and thus not finally being swallowed.

With the rich blood supply, the normal tongue rapidly renews its surface epithelium. Thus, systemic disease and changes in the body as a whole, manifest themselves readily in the tongue. This is due to frequent cell replication, good blood supply and the proximity of micro-organisms in the folds between the papillae of the tongue.

As the tongue shares a common embryological origin with the foregut, lesions in the stomach and intestines may be reflected in the mucous membrane of the tongue, often being more easily visualised there than in more inaccessible examination sites, such as the stomach and intestinal tract.

As the oral cavity is a non-sterile site, and because the growth of such a multitude of micro-organisms is mostly but not completely controlled by the saliva, it is easy to accumulate debris from the micro-organisms, from food and other ingested materials, between the filiform papillae and around the microcrypts present. These, plus a profusion of dead cells, give a so-called 'coating' to the tongue which is rapidly cleaned off by the abrasive action of rough food material. Looking at the tongue becomes an important part of the examination of the patient when thinking about nutritional deficiencies or changes in food habits, as minor deficiencies in micro-nutrients or in the gut lining may show first in such a rapidly replicating surface area. For several decades it has been well-noted by lay health workers that a change from a normal, healthy, high-fibre diet containing large amounts of vegetables and fruit, to convenience foods in a mouth with normal dentition, will change the surface of the tongue. A pink, glistening surface can rapidly change to being coated and white. It is, however, rarely perceived that the coated tongue may be one manifestation of soft, often unhealthy foods with low fibre. The lack of abrasive material in many westernised diets leads to a failure to clean the tongue mechanically. The tongue should not be excessively worn at the edges by normal teeth and gums, and is usually pain-free except when significantly damaged locally by chemical or thermal injury or by systemic disease which alters surface cell replication.

1.1 Development of the tongue

In the very early embryo, the caudal or head part of the embyronic area folds over to enclose the primitive foregut between the amniotic cavity and the primitive pericardium. This foregut is lined on one side by the primitive pericardium and on the other by the developing branchial arches. The area of the subsequent tongue development is associated with the mandibular growth which intervenes between the primitive mouth and the developing thorax. The whole of this development is related to the modification of the six paired branchial arches. These primitive branchial arches are seen in the very earliest invertebrates. They take the form of a series of bars between gill clefts.

Subsequently, with the evolution of earth-living, warm-blooded vertebrates, there was a very rapid evolution of the vertebral arches in the embryo. The jaw-bearing arches are called the mandibular arches, and the next or lower post-mandibular arches go by the name of hyoid arches. The earliest mesenchymae of the branchial region is normally a division between ectoderm and endoderm. The intimate details of how tongue muscle development evolves, especially the change in direction of muscular growth, are unknown. It is generally accepted that the very rich blood supply to the tongue is, in part, derived from the earlier gill cleft arterial requirements for breathing in aquatic evolution.

The primitive mouth area is thus closed underneath by the growth in the floor of the human mandibular arch around from each side. The developing tongue and jaw separate this primitive mouth opening from the pericardium and cardiac development. As the muscle masses migrate from their sites of development, the original innervation persists. The mandibular division of the trigeminal nerve innervates the masculatory musculature of the mandibular arch. The sensory nerves of the tongue for this region are the mandibular branch of the trigeminal nerve (5th) and the chorda tympani branch of the facial nerve (7th), which is the nerve of taste for the anterior region exclusive of the vallate papillae. The lingual branch of the glossopharyngeal nerve (9th) is the nerve of taste and general sensation of the posterior third of the tongue. The superior laryngeal nerve also sends some fine branches to the part of the tongue in front of the epiglottis. The motor function of the tongue is subserved by the hypoglossal nerve (12th nerve).

As Siebert (1985) has pointed out, the tongue doubles its length, width and thickness between birth and adolescence, and the size of the tongue is well-correlated with the size of the head in normal subjects.

1.2 Anatomical features

By convention, the tongue is described as having:

a **root** (posteriorly and beneath)

a **curved dorsal surface** (easily viewed when protruded)

an **inferior** or **ventral surface** (underneath the tip and sides).

The tip and dorsum of the tongue are covered by a mass of filiform papillae interspersed by larger fungiform papillae. Further back is the 'V' shaped defence mechanism of the circumvallate papillae. These more obvious castle-shaped papillae reach the lateral borders of the tongue just in front of the palatoglossal arches. Near here, on the very lateral edge of the tongue, is a small anterior-posterior line of foliate papillae.

It is now accepted that these larger circumvallate papillae and all the other vallate papillae have a specialised function: to prevent the swallowing of a wide distribution of bitter poisonous substances.

The under-surface of the tongue is usually darker, being a purplish-red with prominent venulation. This purple colour can become more marked in the elderly, with thinning of the overlying tissue. The central line of junction of the two halves of the primitive arches in the very early embryo result in a short connecting piece of tissue underneath – the frenulum of the tongue, also sometimes referred to as the frenum. When shorter than usual, this gives rise to so-called 'tongue-tie', and, when lax and long, can lead to an increased mobility of the tongue. On the dorsum the site of fusion may give rise to an island – so-called median rhomboid glossitis. This can sometimes be seen to be reddened to represent an island of glossitis. *Candida* infection in the elderly causing these changes is not usually seen in the young, suggesting controversy regarding a developmental origin (Ullmann & Hoffman, 1981).

1.3 Surface of the tongue

The specialised tasting and sensitive surface feeling functions of the tongue are subserved by the papillae. These functions are learned from birth and during early infancy when most objects are, where possible, explored by the tongue unless too big or too unpleasant! The papillae are really projections or folds of the so-called lamina-propria or cellular basis of the surface. These papillae have been called:

papillae simplices
papillae filiformes
papillae fungiforms
papillae vallate
papillae circumvallate

and are evolved to increase the surface area of the mucous membrane.

The taste buds are more widely scattered than the papillae, which are confined to the anterior two-thirds of the tongue. These taste buds, which have evolved as specialised receptors, are found over the entire dorsum of the tongue (Laverack & Coslens, 1981), and along the sides of the tongue, the epiglottis and the lingual surface of the soft palate. These taste buds are especially concentrated in the vallate papillae (Ferrell & Tsuetaki, 1984). Branches of the 7th (facial) and the 9th (glossopharyngeal) nerves serve these taste receptors.

Between 16 and 96 years of age, the mean epithelial layer undergoes a 30% reduction in thickness. The basal or so-called progenitor cell layer remains the same but the surface layers become progressively thinner with age. The epithelial layer also becomes thinner with age and more so in females than males. This may be one explanation of the more frequent occurrence of glossitis in elderly women. The slow rate of renewing the cells (Scott *et al.*, 1983) is responsible for this loss of thickness.

1.4 Sensory modalities

In early aquatic vertebrates, forms of chemo-receptors are found on the skin in specialised areas. In man, taste sensations derived in the taste receptors distinguish only four main sensations. Zones of special sensitivity appear to exist for sweetness and saltiness at the tip and centre of the tongue, hydrogen ion concentration or acidity at the sides and bitterness mainly around the pharyngeal area. With the gradual sampling of more and more substances after weaning, some tastes can be learned, with some cross-over between groups of receptors in different areas. Only sophisticated statistical analysis of varying strengths of substances allows formal tasting to be carried out. There is no simple relationship of single taste buds to specific tastes.

Adaptation, recruitment and reinforcement can all take place. A simplified schematic diagram presents a consensus view of the most accepted zones or areas.

Animal experiments have always suggested an enlarged sensory representation of the tongue in the post-central gyrus of the brain. An important paper reports accurate mapping of sensory cortical representation in man in 100 patients undergoing craniotomy (Picard & Olivier, 1983). As in animals, there is the same disproportionately large cortical representation of the human tongue in the area just behind the post-central gyrus. Motor representation and sensory tongue responses overlap in this area. There is bilateral representation to a significant degree, but sensory areas are more marked on the dominant hemisphere for speech.

In familial dysautonosmia, which is a rare familial autosomal condition in some Jewish families, swallowing difficulties are associated with lack of development of circumvallate and fungiform papillae, and decreased taste sensation for sweetness and, particularly, bitterness is reported (Gadoth *et al.*, 1982).

Above all, the tongue is a unique feeling instrument. It has the capacity for great plasticity and gives great survival value to the suckling and growing infant. Small hairs, unable to be felt by light touch receptors on the fingers, can easily be distinguished by the tongue. It has exceptional sensitivity, although our understanding of its proprioceptive function is not yet complete.

1.5 Muscles of the tongue

The powerful genioglossus muscle appears to retain its power and force throughout life, although some observers using ultrasound suggest a reduction in volume with age. The striated muscle groups run vertically and intersect the longitudinal musculature. As the posterior muscles are also attached to the somewhat flexible hyoid bone, the tongue is remarkably versatile in volume, shape and, particularly, mobility. Posteriorly in the tongue, the muscle groups of the two halves are bound along the midline, by a fibrous septum.

Nearer the front of the tongue the muscle fibres decussate across the midline and are blended together as they reach not quite to the tip. This large genioglossus muscle, when contracted, draws the tongue forward, protruding the apex between the teeth and flattening the concave dorsal surface. The thinner, strap-like hypoglossus muscle, arising from the hyoid rather than the mandible, draws the tongue downward when it contrasts.

The styloglossus is a small muscle which divides posteriorly to enter the tongue and blend with the longitudinal muscles. It thus draws the tongue backwards and upwards exposing the ventral surface, or underside, on contracting. Tongue muscles are supplied by the hypoglossal or 12th cranial nerve.

1.6 Blood supply of the tongue

The large lingual branches of the external carotid arteries supply a rich network of branches to this most vascular organ. Facial and tonsillar arteries also enter and supply the lingual root of the tongue. The large veins are easily seen on the lateral and ventral surfaces of the tongue. They drain the network of small vascular anastomoses just below the epithelial surface of the tongue.

1.7 Normal tongues of all ages

The tongue in normal, healthy people should be entirely symmetrical with a smooth edge and dorsum, or surface. The surface in good health should be pink and glistening from a free flow of saliva and should protrude easily from the centre of the mouth. The dorsum may show the fine filiform papillae, and occasionally fungiform papillae, but undue prominence of these may suggest early glossitis, especially if pain is present. In the normal tongue the wide variation in colour depends upon minor degrees of coating which itself is largely dependent upon diet.

1.8 Changes in taste

Drugs (such as penicillamine), xerostomia or changes due to radiotherapy (or dry mouth) and changes in zinc metabolism may all lead to changes in taste perception. The following series of photographs show the wide range of appearances of normal tongues from healthy subjects of various races and ages. The tongue surfaces may differ markedly, mainly because of the food choices by these people, although oral hygiene and smoking will also modify the appearance or colour.

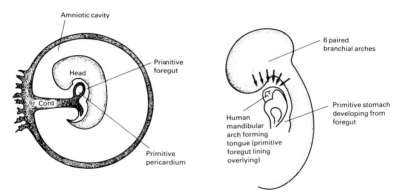

1 Development of the tongue. Simplified drawing of early development of tongue.

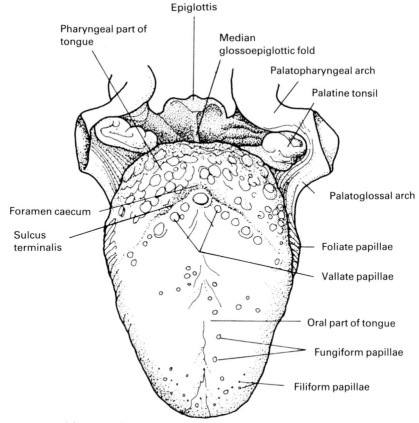

2 Anatomical features of the dorsum of the tongue.

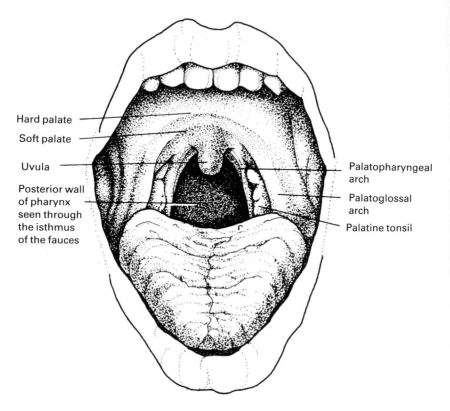

Hard palate

Soft palate

Uvula

Posterior wall
of pharynx
seen through
the isthmus
of the fauces

Palatopharyngeal
arch

Palatoglossal
arch

Palatine tonsil

3 Diagrammatic representation looking towards the fauces.

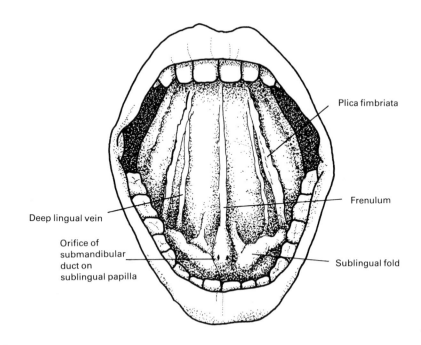

Plica fimbriata

Frenulum

Deep lingual vein

Orifice of
submandibular
duct on
sublingual papilla

Sublingual fold

4 Representation of main anatomical features of ventral surface of tongue.

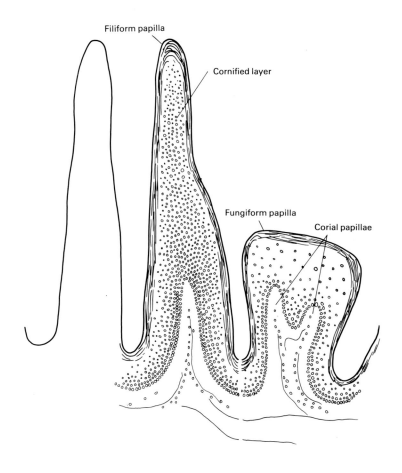

5   Simplified features of the main papillae of the tongue.

6 Filiform papillae highlighted in a cleaned, normal elderly tongue.

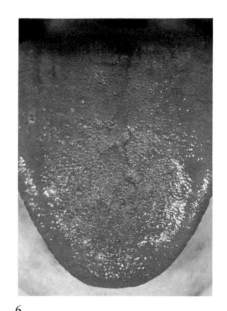

7 Close-up view of normal filiform papillae in a healthy older child.

6

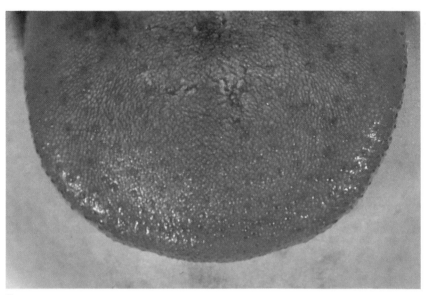

7

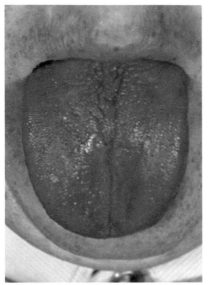

8

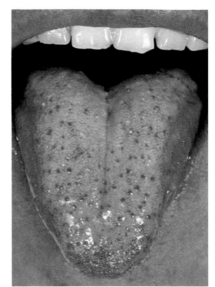

9

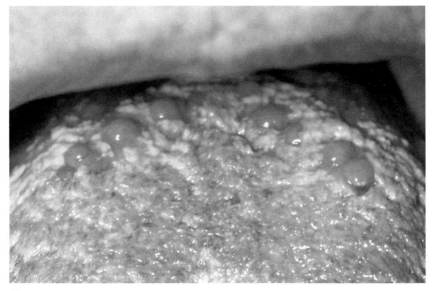

10

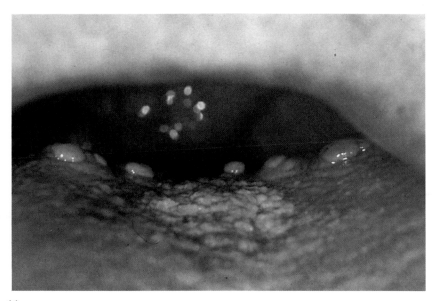

11

8   Elderly man with slight superficial glossitis (from drugs) and partial loss of filiform papillae. Fungiforms show well on the right.

9   Coated tongue in a Polynesian with pneumonia, the coating emphasises fungiform papillae.

10   An 81-year-old woman hospitalised with diabetic complications. Mouth candidiasis and coating of tongue emphasises the circumvallate papillae.

11   Enlarged circumvallate papillae well visualised.

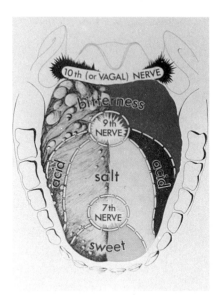

12 Sensory modalities. A diagramatic representation of taste distribution on the tongue.

12

13 Diagrammatic schema of the sensory representation of the tongue in the cerebral cortex. Note these very large areas and the fact that both sensory and motor functions cross over into their opposite areas. Motor representation creeps into the sensory cortex and some senory fibres finish up in the motor area.

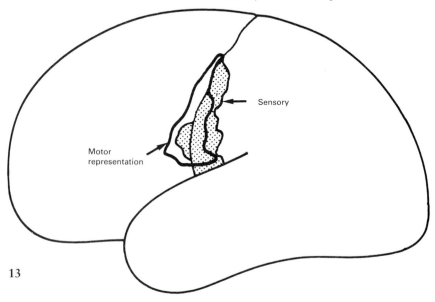

13

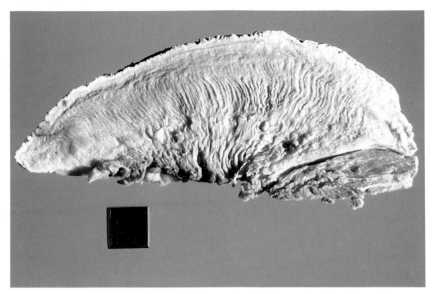

14

14 Longitudinal cross-section from an autopsy specimen showing bulk of tongue muscles from an elderly female.

15 Transverse cross-section of the tongue, also from a recent autopsy specimen, to show network of muscle fibres in different directions to give plasticity to the tongue section across the tongue near the 'root' and midway in the tongue.

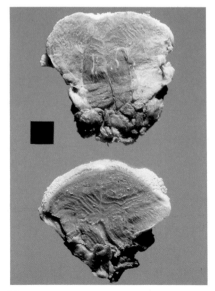

15

27

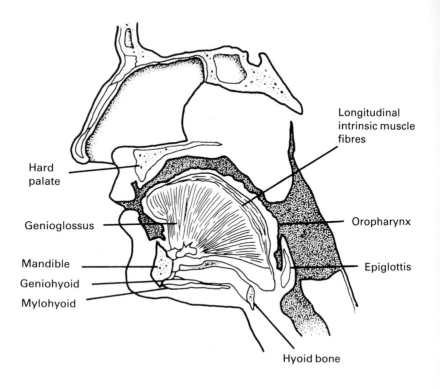

16 Semi-diagrammatic representation of main muscle groups.

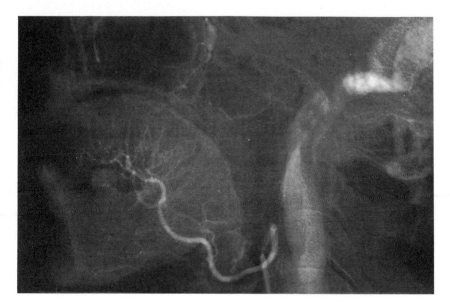

17 Angiogram of the tongue to show the great vascularity from the many vertical branches.

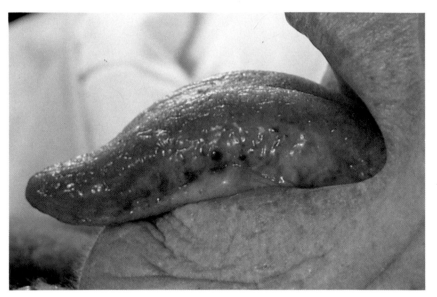

18

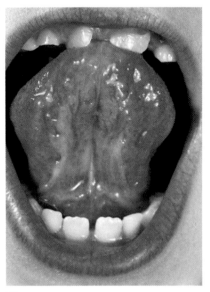

19

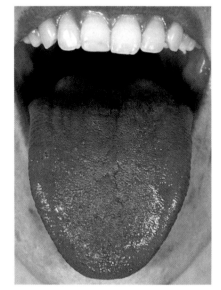

20

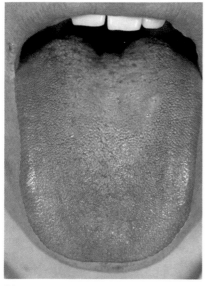

21

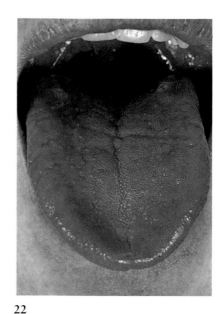

22

18 Venous return from the tongue shown clearly in 96-year-old woman with view from the lateral side of the tongue.

19 Main ventral veins of the tongue well seen in young normal subject.

20 Normal healthy 22-year-old, non-smoking, semi-vegetarian, female medical student.

21 Normal healthy 21-year-old Chinese male student, non-smoking, semi-westernised diet.

22 Normal healthy 30-year-old Caucasian female vegetarian with very clean tongue.

23 Normal young semi-vegetarian Indian male, living in a westernised environment.

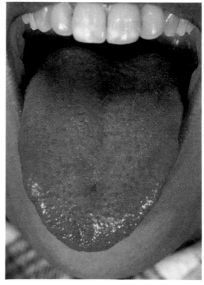

23

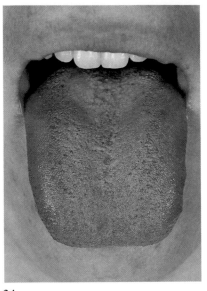 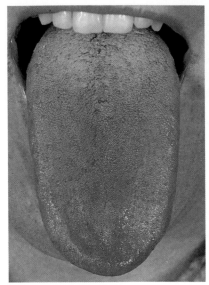

24

25

24 Normal healthy 21-year-old male smoker, eating a westernised diet.

25 Normal healthy non-smoking 22-year-old male, normal westernised diet.

26 Normal healthy 36-year-old female.

27 Normal healthy meat-eating male clerk, an occasional smoker.

28 Normal 40-year-old male doctor, non-smoker.

29 Normal 21-year-old Eurasian male, non-smoker, westernised diet.

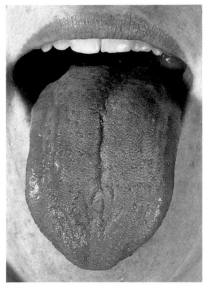

26

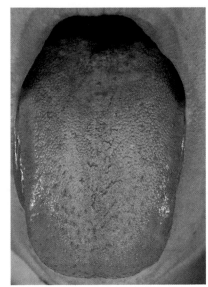

27

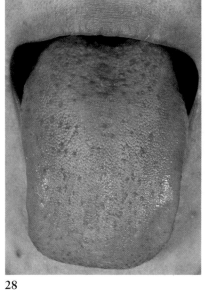

28

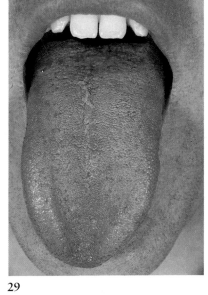

29

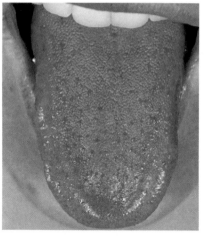

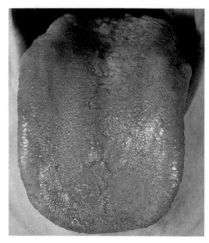

30

31

30   Normal healthy 25-year-old female physiotherapist, non-smoker.

31   Normal healthy 30-year-old married female, Australasian diet, non-smoker.

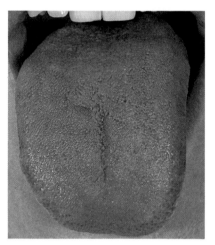

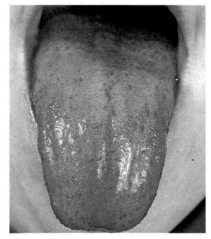

32

33

32   Normal healthy 14-year-old female, normal diet, non-smoker.

33   Normal healthy 5-year-old female of mixed racial background.

34

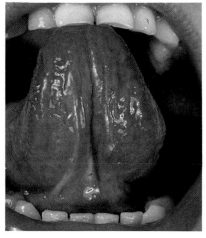 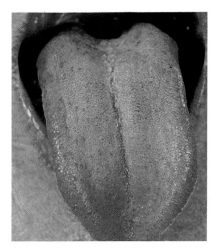

34   35

34 Good view of the ventral surface of the tongue in a healthy European child of 7 years. Note glistening appearance of free saliva flow and normal frenum.

35 Normal healthy 60-year-old physician, non-smoking, normal European diet.

References

Ferrell F., Tsuetaki T. Regeneration of taste buds after surgical excision of human vallate papill. *Exp Neurol* 1984, **83**, (2), 429-445.

Gadoth N., Margalith D.O.V., Schlein N. *et al. Johns Hopkins Med J* 1982, **151**, 298-301.

Laverack M.S., Coslens D.J. (Eds). *Sense Organs,* 1st edn. Blackie, Glasgow, 1981, pp88-99.

Picard C. O. Olivier A. Sensory cortical tongue. Representation in man. *J Neurosurg* 1983, **59**, 781-789.

Scott J., Valentine J.A., St Hill C.A. *et al.* A quantitative histological analysis of the effects of age and sex on human lingual epithelium. *J Biol Buccale* 1983, **11**(4), 303-315.

Siebert J.R. A morphometric study of normal and abnormal fetal to childhood tongue size. *Arch Oral Biol* 1985, **30**(5), 433-440.

Ullmann W., Hoffman M. Glossitis rhombica mediana. A study of 4422 dermatologic patients. *Hautarzt* 1981, **32**(11), 571-574.

Williams P.L., Warwick R. (Eds). *Grays Anatomy*, 36th edn. Churchill Livingstone, London, 1980.

Chapter 2
Examination of the Mouth and Tongue

This guide is for the non-specialist and for those who have limited time to examine the mouth. Thus, detailed methods of more specialised examination of the gingiva and soft tissues of the mouth are more properly the domain of the oral medicine specialist or dental practitioner. Clearly, however, the health worker who looks at the tongue in a routine examination should proceed to a more detailed inspection of other areas of the mouth and tongue if any changes excite curiosity.

Most people presenting to primary health care systems expect the pulse to be felt and the outstretched tongue to be examined. A major textbook for medical students on clinical methods published in 1973 (Tumulty) devoted only 10 lines out of over 270 pages to the tongue, and there are only five lines in a popular 338-page book on clinical diagnosis (Buckingham, 1979). By 1982, however, a small volume for the British clinician gave 10 pages to the tongue (Bouchier & Morris, 1982).

The tongue should always be inspected during general clinical interviews by health professionals. A request to open the mouth and protrude the tongue will also include observation of the dorsum and, on phonation, the hard and soft palates can be seen in good light. Clinical competence should be built on repetitive practice of skills, together with intellect, wisdom and, above all, curiosity (Richards, 1986). Any abnormalities should arouse this curiosity but small changes need to be observed more carefully.

Observation of the dorsum of the tongue is ideally carried out in natural sunlight or under an angled lamp. So-called 'clinical' or pocket torches recommended for medical students and house staff are useless.

Any abnormality on the edges or the dorsum of the tongue alerts the health worker to the need for a better and more careful clinical look at all areas of the mouth and gingiva, including the ventral or under-surface of the tongue. White patches are abnormal but the throat stick or spatula or better still a dental mirror can be useful in removing adherent material.

Swabs and a local anaesthetic need to be at hand. A warmed laryngeal mirror for the back of the tongue and rubber gloves are needed in palpation within the mouth due to potential danger from infections from suspected immuno-deficiency virus (HIV) or Hepatitis B. Unusual or opportunistic infections may also gain entry to the mouth through tongue or gingival lesions

Table 1 Smelling the breath

Odours on breath	Association likely	Possible findings
Sweet, volatile, 'pear-drop'-like	Acetone	In fasting or calorie deficiency (especially children) Insulin deficiency (diabetes mellitus) Fever and increased metabolic states
Alcohol-like, stale aromas	Alcohol	Alcohol abuse or alcoholism Especially in accident victims Look for spider naevi Lattice of new vessels on malar areas, conjunctival yellowness, palmar erythema, sweating
Mouse-like	Candidiasis (oro-pharangeal)	Steroid therapy, antibiotic use and diabetes mellitus
Purulent and offal sweetness	Bronchiectasis	Productive cough (repetitive), clubbing of nails at nail folds Possible slight cyanosis
Pungent, musty, ammoniacal: slightly old eggs	Fetor hepaticus (mercaptans, and nitrogenous compounds)	Sallow skin, dulled consciousness, 'flapping' tremor
Metallic and purulent, slightly sweet offal odours	Gum infections	Neglected and broken teeth Heavy drug therapy (antibiotics anti-cancer drugs) 'smoker's' fingers I.V. drug sites along arm veins
Uraemic breath	Renal failure and nitrogenous retention	Sallow, pigmented and anaemic skin. Brown lines on nails, urea 'snow'
Unpleasant faeculent and pyogenic odours	Sinusitis and nasal malignancy, necrosis (e.g. Wegener's)	Febrile and ill patients with weight loss

in debilitated patients, drug addicts and in oncology or immunosuppressed patients.

Smelling the breath should be part of the careful clinical examination of any seriously ill person. For unconscious patients it is mandatory!

The sense of smell is the Cinderella of the senses in western industrialised society but was essential to survival in primitive mankind. Repeatedly practising the close smelling of the breath, as illustrated, will improve the ability to know when abnormal smells are present. These can arise from the mouth or be volatile substances excreted through the lungs.

When the mouth is open and the tongue is being examined, we have also found it useful to spend 20 seconds running the index finger around the upper and lower teeth to estimate the degree of sharpness. Malocclusions can be a cause of sharp teeth, and excessively sharpened teeth are often associated with internal or exogenous stresses.

36 Visual inspection of the dorsum of the tongue in good sunlight near a window.

37 Examination of the dorsum of the tongue by good torchlight.

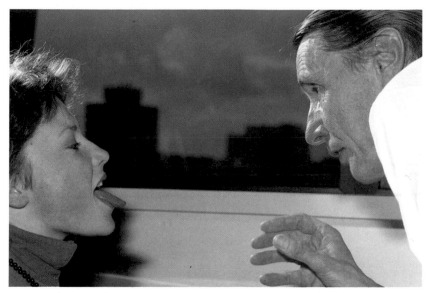

36

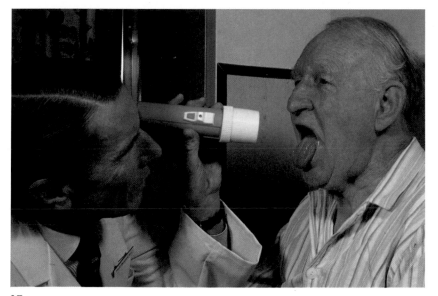

37

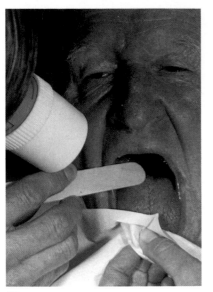 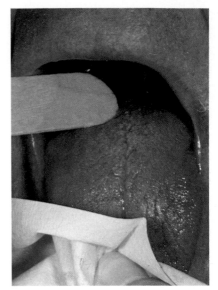

38   39

38-41 Further examination of the tongue using a spatula, which is also being used for full examination of the mouth, including the ventral or under-surface of the tongue.

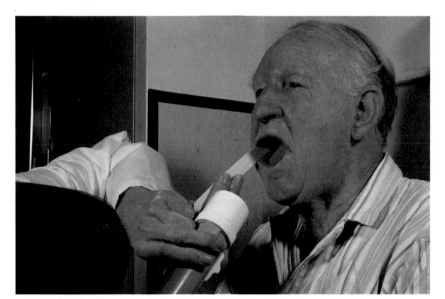

40

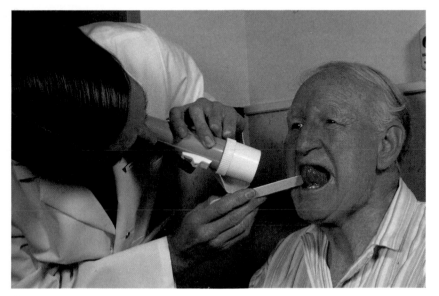

41

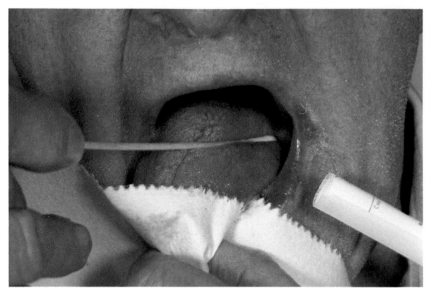

42

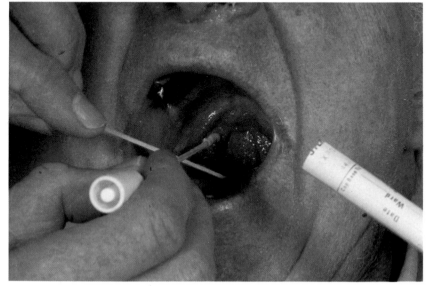

43

42

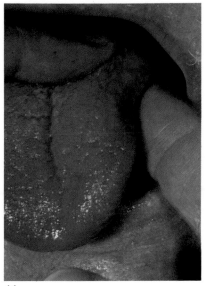
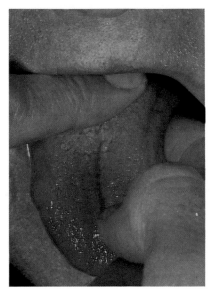

44 **45**

42 and 43 Taking microbiological swabs from the dorsum and ventral surface of the tongue. The same technique is used when firmly scraping the surface of the tongue and when taking other hypheal forms of *Candidiasis*.

44 and 45 Palpation of the tongue using both hands to identify abnormalities in the depth of the muscle bulk or root.

References

Bouchier I.A.D., Morris J.S. *Clinical Skills*, 2nd edn. W.B. Saunders, London, 1982.
Buckingham W.B. *A Primer of Clinical Diagnosis*. 2nd edn Harper & Row, 1979, p47.
Richards P. Clinical competence and curiosity. *Br Med J* 1986, **292**, 1481-1482.
Tumulty P.A. *The Effective Clinician. His Methods and Approach to Diagnosis and Care*, 1st edn W.B. Saunders, Philadelphia, 1973, p70.

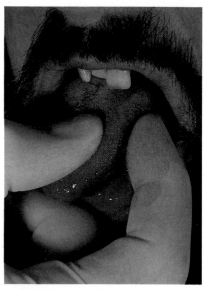

46 Using protective rubber gloves, bimanual palpation of suspected Kaposi sarcoma in AIDS antibody positive young man.

47 Inspection of the tongue and mouth is incomplete without carefully smelling the breath.

46

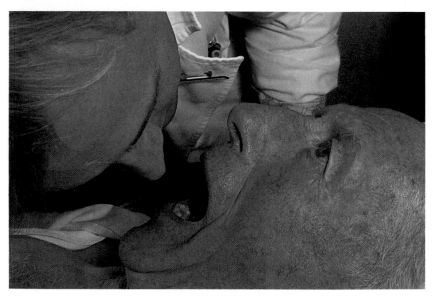

47

Chapter 3
Dehydration, saliva and the tongue

A high proportion of people referred to oral medicine specialists for dry mouth do, in fact, have auto-immune disease of the salivary glands. This is especially so in patients who have Sjögren's syndrome and sarcoidosis. In chronic dry mouth syndromes papillary atrophy may begin to appear. In primary care medicine acute 'in the field' infections are more common. Thus, illnesses which increase the metabolic rate may also lead to an increased respiratory rate with mouth breathing. The dorsal surface of the tongue becomes parched. Surface dryness of the tongue is, therefore, a poor guide to the percentage water loss or the actual degree of total body dehydration. In normal young adults the changes in skin turgor are a late sign of dehydration. In those over 65 years increasing looseness of the skin can be mistaken for dehydration.

For non-specialists in the area and 'field-workers' it is recommended that the sides of the tongue and the frothiness of the saliva under the tongue be examined. This is in no way a simple or even scientific test but when the dorsum of the tongue is parched in mouth breathing, such additional information may be helpful. As many clinical measurements as possible should be done to assess the degree of dehydration. The following should all be used together in acute medical disorders:

History of thirst and a low urine output (as in uncontrolled diabetes mellitus).

Rising pulse and falling blood pressure may be useful in acute dehydration.

Top of venous pressure wave with head downwards (indicates reduction in 5 litres of total fluid volume if the top of the column does not become visible).

How easily does the finger slide in and out under the dry tongue?

Eyeball tension fluctuation by safe, light touch, rocking technique shown (combined ECF and circulating fluid volume)?

Turgor of skin in at least two standard sites can indicate some possible reduction in total body water.

Osmoreceptors and thirst are activated with a 2% fall in osmolality, and clinical dehydration should be detected with a 5% fall in total extra-cellular water (total body water = 60% of body weight; ECF approximately one-third of total water or approximately 15 litres, of which 5 to 5.5 is total blood volume) (Stein, 1983).

Laboratory tests (Krupp *et al.*, 1979) such as a changing plasma urea, packed cell volume and osmolality at intervals and a central venous pressure line and manometer (Eknoyan, 1981) may be needed in severe and acute dehydration.

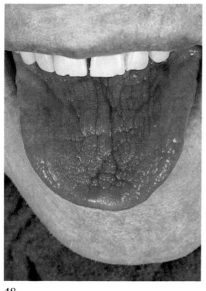 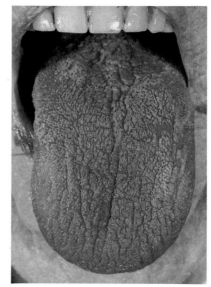

48   49

48   78-year-old-diabetic with increasing tolbutamide failure and admitted to hospital with diabetic ketoacidosis and moderate dehydration.

49   Elderly man with repeated vomiting from small bowel obstruction. Coated tongue has resulted from no food intake. Note also cyanosis of tongue and lip edges. The large tongue when dehydrated suggested the possibility of hypothyroidism, later confirmed by high TSH levels.

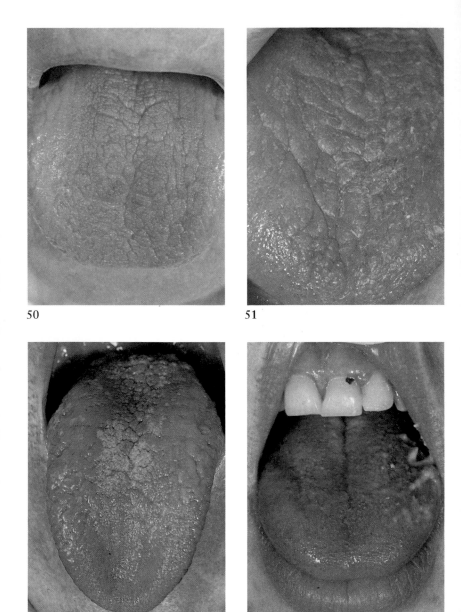

50

51

52

53

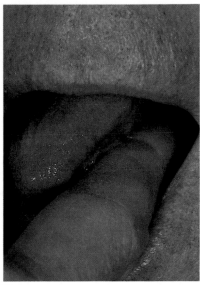

54

50 Pale, elderly, retired man with chronic kidney failure, anaemia and dehydration.

51 Elderly woman admitted to hospital with chronic diarrhoea. Measuring packed cell volume, electrolytes and osmolality confirm 15% dehydration.

52 Dry tongue from mouth-breathing, secondary to emphysema. Laboratory and clinical measurements did not confirm dehydration. Note early cyanosis.

53 Tenacious frothy saliva suggests early dehydration in young female on high diuretic dosage.

54 How easily does the finger slide in and out under the tongue? A sometimes useful clinical test for dehydration.

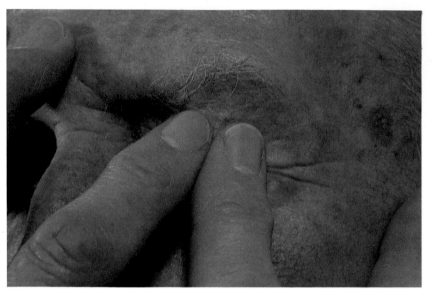

55

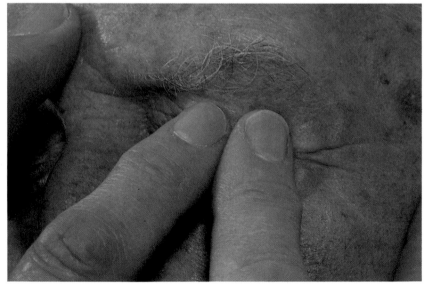

56

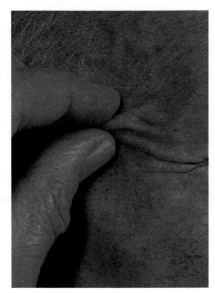

57

55 and 56 Eyeball tension as a good test of dehydration is being measured by lightly fluctuating pressure of the two index fingers on the eyeball. As seen, rocking movements from one finger to the other help the detection of the softness of the globe.

57 Skin turgor or the amount of tissue water should be measured in at least two sites on the body, here measured in the temple area.

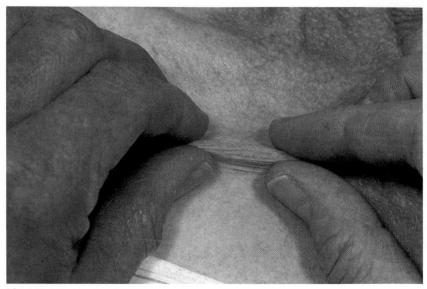

58

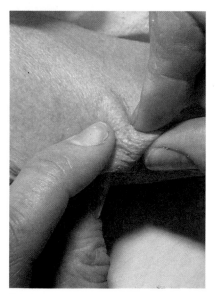

59

58 and 59 Skin turgor being measured by pinching the skin at one standardised site just beneath the scapula and another close to the elbow.

60 and 61 Central venous pressure can be measured by an intravenous catheter and manometer or more simply by tilting the foot of the bed upwards 15 or 20 degrees so that the patient is lying with the head sloping downwards. The jugular venous system in the neck may remain empty when there is marked dehydration and volume depletion.

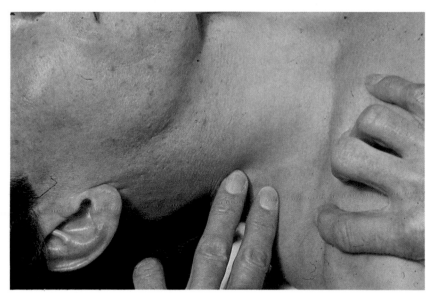

60

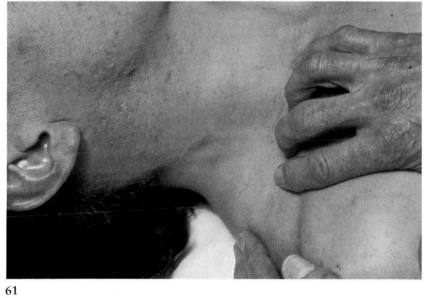

61

53

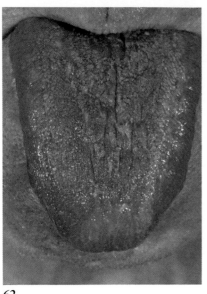

62 Very dehydrated, terminally ill old woman who refused all fluids.

62

References

Eknoyan G. *Medical Procedures Manual*, 1st edn. Year Book, Chicago, 1981, pp163-181.

Hope R.A., Longmore J.M. *Oxford Handbook of Clinical Medicine*, Oxford University Press, Oxford, 1985, p.562.

Krupp M.A., Sweet N.J., Jawatz E., *et al*. Fluid and electrolyte balance. In: *Physician's Handbook*, 19th edn. Lange Medical Publications, Los Altos, California, 1979, pp475-477.

Stein J.H. *Internal Medicine*, 1st edn. Little Brown, Boston, 1983.

Chapter 4

Large Tongues

Rarely do patients come to medical attention complaining of the increasing size of the tongue. When this occurs, the diagnosis is nearly always acromegaly or hypothyroidism. Lowering of thyroid hormones in the blood is a relatively common condition whereas acromegaly is a rare one. We have seen only two acromegalic patients out of a series of about 40 who have a tongue too large to be comfortably accommodated in the mouth. Larger than normal tongues have been reported in Down's syndrome or Trisomy 21, possibly emphasised by the hypotonia present but often the tongue is in fact found to be of normal size, the mouth being smaller than usual, although the margins of the tongue are sometimes scalloped. Criteria for measuring tongue size are poorly developed and should relate to cranial measurements. Thus, if the typical facial appearance of Down's syndrome is absent, a likely diagnosis is acromegaly (confirmed by raised serum growth hormone after meals) or, more likely, hypothyroid disease. Rare causes (Hart, 1973) of a large tongue are: haemangiomata in the body of the tongue, muscular hypertrophy or amyloidosis with tongue involvement. The last is a rare disorder but well-documented (Beiser *et al.*, 1980; Yamaguchi *et al.*, 1982; Van der Wal *et al.*, 1984).

Also reported are enlarged tongues in the rare Opitz-Kaveggia disease with mid-face anomalies, and hemihypertrophy of skeletal muscles.

The excellent review by Siebert (1985) of childhood tongue size is based on a morphometric study of tongue sizes measured in cadavers from foetus to 10 years of age.

We have not seen a very large tongue without some recognisable pathological state present, except in totally and habitually edentulous patients where the tongue appears to spread outwards between the alveolar ridges.

Lastly, trauma to the tongue, with haematoma formation not immediately visible, may lead to enlargement of the tongue.

Table 2 Large tongues

Diagnosis	Frequency	Mechanisms
In young		
Cretinism	Extremely rare (except in mountain and volcanic areas)	Lack of thyroid hormone (congenital)
Down's syndrome	Commonest	Trisomy 21
Congenital macroglossia	Very rare	Abnormality with or without chromosome 16
Adults		
Hypothyroidism	Common	Lack of thyroid hormone
Edentulous	Various ethnic and national groups	Tongue grows to fill space in mouth
Acromegaly	Rare	Growth hormone excess
Amyloid Local general	Extremely rare Very rare	Accumulation of amyloid material locally or microscopically throughout tongue
Tumours	Rare	Deep or ventral tumours
Acute glossitis and angio-neurotic oedema	Less common but can be life-threatening	Insect bites Bee stings Acute thermal or Chemical reactions
Crohn's and gut diseases	Very uncommon	Swelling and hypertrophied areas due to chronic inflammation

63   Classical large fissured tongue due to Down's syndrome (Trisomy 21).

64   Down's syndrome male with a large tongue. It is unusual to see such a small number of fissures but there is a coexistant median rhomboid glossitis present.

65   Congenital cretinism can give large tongues in small children. Thyroid treatment reduces the size, but omission of therapy over some months led to a deterioration back to a large tongue in this young man.

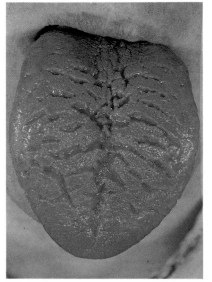

63

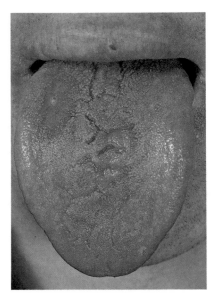

64

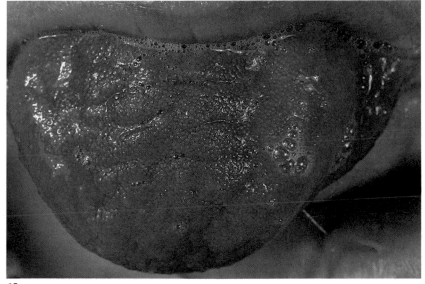

65

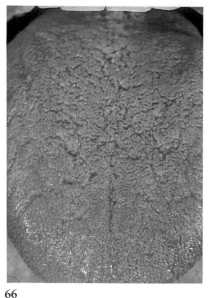 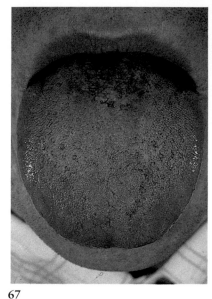

66   Macroglossia can be congenital without Trisomy 21. Here an unusually large arm E16 chromosome (see Chapter 17) is associated with a very big tongue.

67   An older man with severe undiagnosed hypothyroidism. Hypothyroidism is undoubtedly the commonest cause of a large tongue in adults.

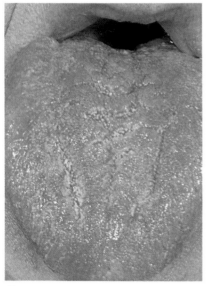

68

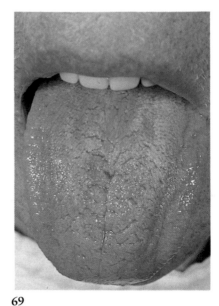

69

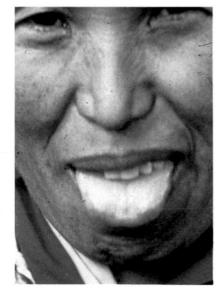

70

68 Hypothryoid tongue with anaemia, B_{12} deficiency is by far the most common association. Gastric atrophy unlikely (because no obvious smoothness or chronic atrophic glossitis of tongue edges).

69 Hypothyroidism secondary to goitre surgery several years before, in this older Chinese male.

70 A large coated tongue in this colourful Nepalese male treated for cretinism.

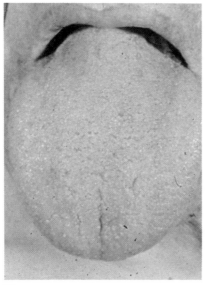

71

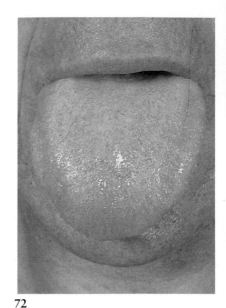

72

71 An elderly male with severe acromegaly. The large tongue was later the cause of death before treatment was fully effective.

72 The large pale tongue of a mildly acromegalic male. Some early hypertensive heart failure and early pulmonary oedema were also present, as frequently occurs in elderly acromegalics.

73 Classical 'furrowing' of the brow due to soft tissue over-growth in an acromegalic man.

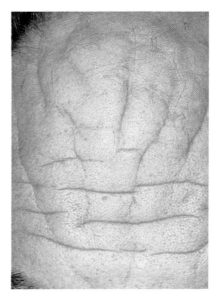

73

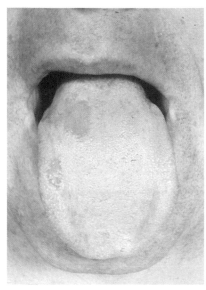

74 A comparatively rapid tongue enlargement in a young male with acromegaly. Also shown is an early geographic tongue.

75 The large tongue of acromegaly just seen behind the teeth of a young woman. The teeth are spread apart because of growth hormone-induced over-growth of jaw ridges.

74

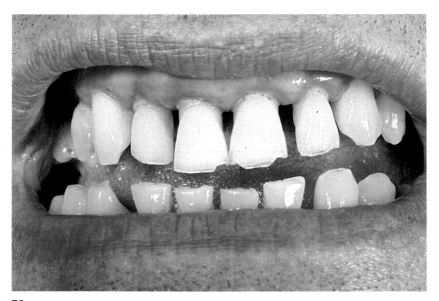

75

76 'Giant' young Chinese male with growth hormone excess.

77 Gross coating of the tongue and also erosions of upper lip in an acromegalic with diabetes. Scalloped tongue edges have resulted from the growth pressure of the large tongue on the inner surfaces of the teeth.

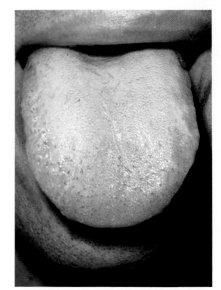

76

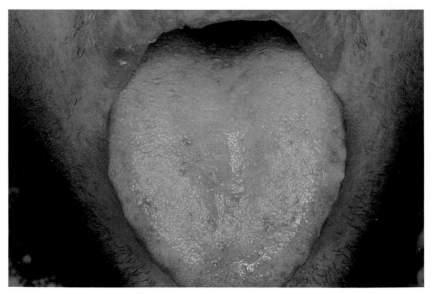

77

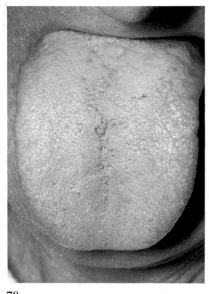

78

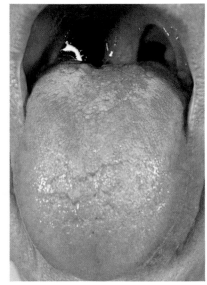

79

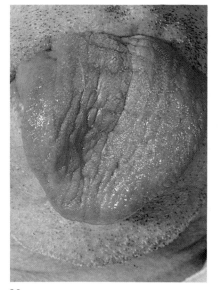

80

78 A permanent edentulous state in this middle-aged male smoker has led to the compensatory growth in size of the tongue. As he does not own any dentures, the tongue has become quite gross to fill the space which would normally have been taken up by teeth!

79 An elderly man whose large tongue appears to be related to the fact that he has been devoid of either teeth or dentures for many years.

80 Some local amyloid accumulation on the right side of the tongue. Amyloid also present in spleen and liver.

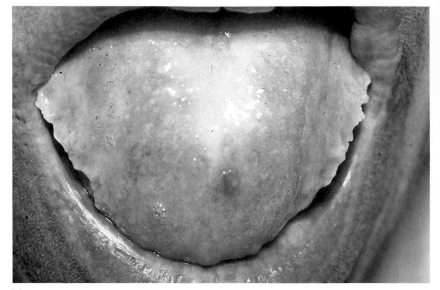

81

81 Very woody, diffusively enlarged tongue in a general amyloidosis in a negroid man.

82 Elderly male presented with enlarged tongue caused by a deeply placed tumour. A later biopsy showed squamous cell carcinoma.

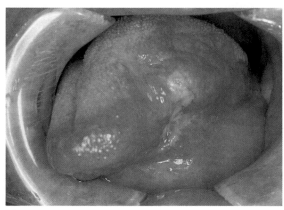

82

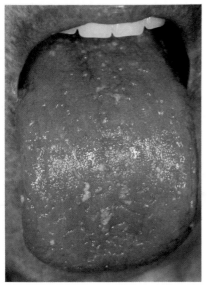
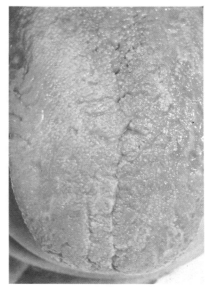

83   84

83 Acute general glossitis, very large tongue secondary to phenytoin hyperplasia, more usually affecting the gingivae, not shown here.

84 Large acromegalic tongue from 39-year-old woman showing marked coating of the tongue secondary to depression and failure to eat. There is a little scalloping on the right edge. The hypertrophy of the tongue highlights the fissures and enlarged fungiform papillae over the base.

References

Beiser M., Messer G., Samuel J. *et al.* Amyloidosis of Waldeyer's ring. A clinical and ultrastructural report. *Acta Otolaryngol* (Stockholm) 1980, **89**(5-6), 562-569.

Hart F.D., (Ed). *French's Index of Differential Diagnosis*, 10th edn. John Wright, Bristol, 1973, p.769.

Siebert J.R. A morphometric study of normal and abnormal fetal to childhood tongue size. *Arch Oral Biol* 1985, **30**, 5, 433-440.

Van der Wal N., Henzen-Logmans S., Van der Kwast W.A.M. *et al.* Amyoidosis of the tongue: A clinical and post-mortem study. *J Oral Path* 1984, **13**, 632-639.

Yamaguchi A., Nasu M., Esaki Y. *et al.* Amyloid deposits in the aged tongue: A post-mortem study of 107 individuals over 60 years of age. *J Oral Path* 1982, **11**(3), 237-244.

Chapter 5
Small Tongues

In the young, a very small tongue is often associated with craniofacial or extracranial anomalies. Although the exact mechanism of the development is not clear, maldevelopment of the branchial arches early in embryogenesis between 4 and 6 weeks of gestation appears to be responsible for a hypoplastic or small tongue (Oulis & Thornton, 1982). Small tongues in infancy are seen in:

    congenital small mandible syndromes
    lingual hypoplasia
    Pierre-Robin syndrome
    congenital facial diplegia
    aglossia adactylia
    other rare developmental disorders (McCarthy & Shklar, 1980; Anderson
        & Kissane 1984).

Only in wasting disease and severe dehydration does the tongue shrink slightly. In increasing age the normal tongue is preserved from the wasting seen in other general muscles. Pseudo-bulbar palsy and bulbar palsies from motor neurone disease are exceptions.

Pseudo-bulbar palsy is the *commonest cause* of small tongue in the elderly in western societies. Repeated small strokes in the capsular area may lead to an increasing degree of bilateral pyramidal tract involvement. In the condition of pseudo-bulbar palsy there is a small spastic tongue, positive jaw and snout 'jerks', and very brisk deep tendon reflexes bilaterally. In pseudo-bulbar palsies, the tongue is wasted and spastic but does not fasciculate in the mouth. For both a fasciculating and wasting tongue the 12th cranial nerve nucleus is involved in repeated vertebro-basilar insufficiency, or a degeneration of brain-stem nuclei as part of motor neurone disease occurs along the course of the 12th nerve.

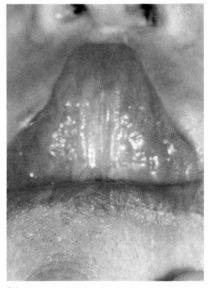

85

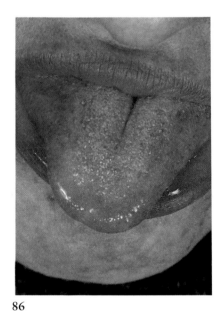

86

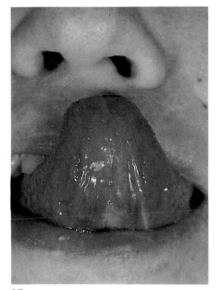

87

85 Congenital small mandible and intellectual handicap with relative microglossia. No chromosomal abnormality was found.

86 Congenital hypoglossia in the 'cri du chat' syndrome.

87 Lingual hypoplasia. No chromosomal abnormalities were found but mild intellectual impairment was present.

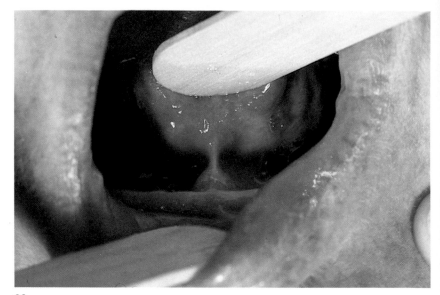

88

88 Congenital short lingual frenum of the tongue with some microglossia.

89 Small tongue maximally pushed out. Mobility affected by short frenum. Note also mild medication-induced glossitis in this 9-year-old male.

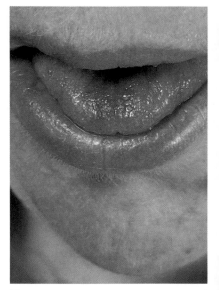

89

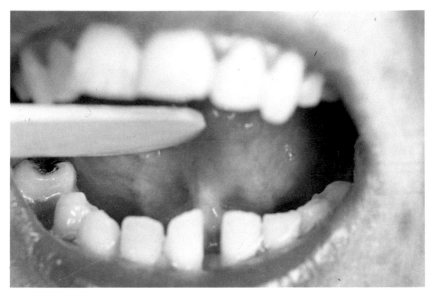

90

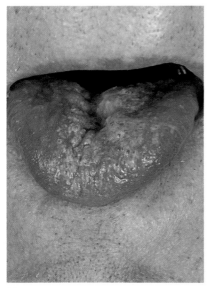

91

90 Teenage female with small tongue unable to be protruded because of abnormally short thick frenum.

91 Bilateral spasticity of tongue prevents protrusion and suggests a thinned and wasted small tongue.

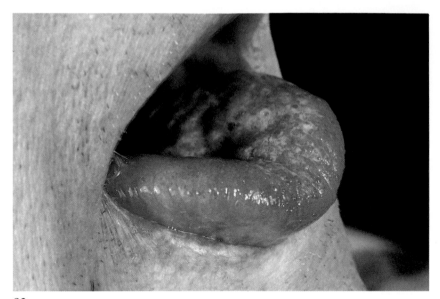

92

92 Lateral view of the same 75-year-old man as in **91**.

93 Small tongue in 56-year-old male. Congenital cause unknown. A slightly marked median fissure, with normal limits, is also present.

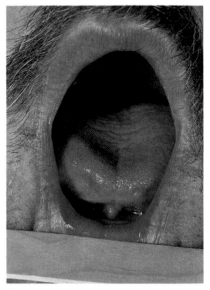

93

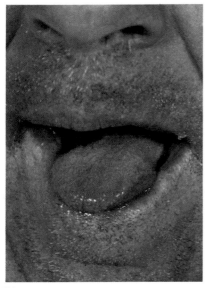 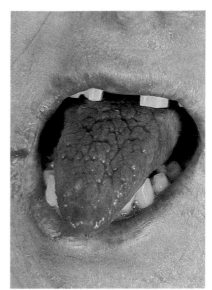

94   95

94   Underdeveloped so called 'mid-face syndrome' where maldevelopment has led to a congenitally small tongue in a 46-year-old male.

95   Atrophic dry mucosa with atrophy of filiforms in a 54-year-old female on multiple medication for hypertension. Bilateral pyramidal tract damage leading to reduction in size of tongue with spasticity. Note small right-sided papilloma.

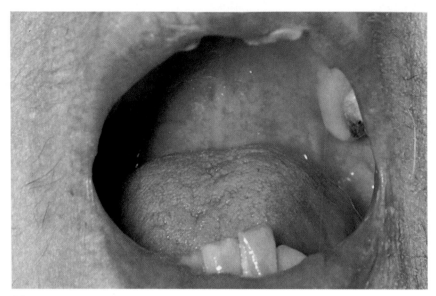

96

96   An elderly female with wasted and shrunken tongue unable to be protruded from the mouth due to bilateral small strokes, and 12th nerve involvement because of bilateral upper motor neurone lesions.

References

Anderson W.A.D., Kissane J.M. *Pathology*, 8th edn. C.V. Mosby, St Louis, 1984, Vol 2, Ch 29.

McCarthy P.L., Shklar G. *Diseases of the Oral Mucosa*, 2nd edn. Lea & Febiger, Philadelphia, 1980, pp77-82.

Oulis C.J., Thornton J.B. Severe congenital hypoglossia and micrognathia with other multiple birth defects. *J Oral Path* 1982, **11**(4), 276-282.

Chapter 6
Coatings of the Tongue

'The layman frequently attaches great weight to the surface appearance of the tongue and may readily develop obsessions about its cleanliness and the significance of any real or imagined changes.'

This quotation from a widely used student textbook published in 1986 (McLeod & Munro) misses the major point that observation of the surface of the tongue is a major exercise for all primary health workers in:

developing the accuracy of their powers of observation;
developing an ability to decide on limits of the degrees of normal or, more properly, good health;
whether the observer is alert enough to decide that deviations from normal are present, and then to ask why.

It is well accepted that an unduly coated tongue is found in heavy smokers, mouth breathers, and those who do not use their dentures. Coated tongues are also seen in those habitually on soft foods (Bomford *et al.*, 1975). The growth of the tips of the filiform papillae allows greater opportunity for collection of debris, dead cells and bacteria in the spaces between the papillae (McCarthy & Shklar, 1980). In evolving omnivorous *Homo sapiens*, the uncooked food was hard, rough and fibrous. As it was repeatedly chewed, it sheared off longer filiform papillae and, by sheer mechanical effects, cleaned the surface of the tongue.

The following views are clearly not proven but are a major hypothetical basis for deductions drawn from more than 20 years of daily clinical observations in routine medical practice.

Today, people who live in a pre-industrial manner (as in the isolated pacific atolls or in Central Java), usually continue to eat largely fibrous vegetables, grains and fruit with some root vegetables such as yams. Protein may be derived from some stringy or tough meat (such as free-running pigs or chickens) or occasionally fish. Such traditional diets normally give healthy pink tongues.

Our food is now more processed, not by the upper gastrointestinal tract but by the increasing use of fossil fuels and factories. It is believed that the types of food eaten in western societies have changed more markedly over the period of recorded scientific observations than have our own teeth and tongue. This is too short a period for natural adaptation or evolution to take place (Beaven & Easton, 1974).

It is now also well accepted by all international advisory bodies that a broad diversity of foods should be a general principle of nutrition. There is also increasing emphasis on high-fibre diets, which also provide a cleansing effect on the tongue. But speed and convenience dictate that we all eat more processed grains as bread or biscuits, vegetables as convenience foods and meats as grain-fed packages. In the middle ages, teeth were often worn to the gums by 40 years of age due to the abrasion of normal food. Today it is rare to see teeth worn down by this age in westernised societies.

Thus, a coated tongue is *not normal*. It may be merely due to fasting for one or two days, as occurs compulsorily in many severe illnesses and high fevers. In the normal ambulant person a coated tongue may be a sign of poor or neglected health. Smoking inevitably leads to a permanent light coat on the tongue, while heavy smoking of cigarettes, pipes or cigars produces dark staining posteriorly. Heavy coatings of the tongue occur in otherwise healthy people who have ill-fitting dentures. It is seldom appreciated that complete dentures need to be remoulded every 5 years. Otherwise, a slowly developing mismatch between rigid artificial dentures and changing gum shape means that high-fibre foods are avoided. In our studies of 200 elderly New Zealand hospital patients a standard timed hard-biscuit eating test showed these older people with upper and lower dentures had only 5-8% the efficiency of younger and middle-aged full mouth dentate people, and there was a 100% incidence of tongue coating. Thus, tongue coatings can suggest current or future ill-health.

The pictures in this chapter show examples of:

'dietary' coatings of the tongue;
thin and heavy coatings;
hairy tongues;
coatings from other causes.

Flow diagram for non-specialised health workers after observing a coated tongue

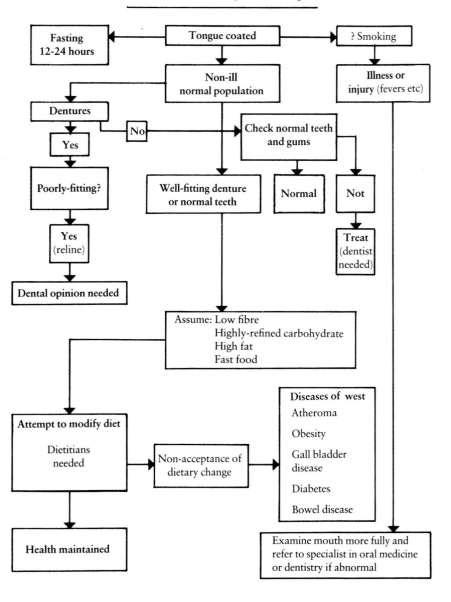

Tongue coated

Fasting 12-24 hours

? Smoking

Non-ill normal population

Illness or injury (fevers etc)

Dentures

No

Check normal teeth and gums

Yes

Poorly-fitting?

Well-fitting denture or normal teeth

Normal

Not

Yes (reline)

Treat (dentist needed)

Dental opinion needed

Assume: Low fibre
Highly-refined carbohydrate
High fat
Fast food

Attempt to modify diet

Dietitians needed

Non-acceptance of dietary change

Diseases of west
Atheroma
Obesity
Gall bladder disease
Diabetes
Bowel disease

Health maintained

Examine mouth more fully and refer to specialist in oral medicine or dentistry if abnormal

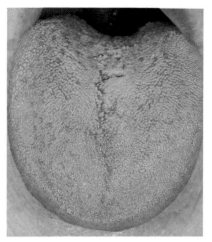

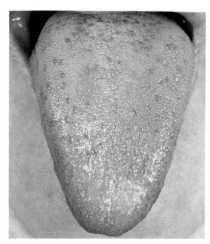

97

98

97 49-year-old male with mild tongue coating secondary to a recent dietary change and avoidance of high-fibre foods. As he is an ex-smoker with documented lung disease this may account for his mild cyanosis.

98 Mild coating of tongue secondary to low-fibre foods. Note marked fungiform papillae over the root or posterior part of the tongue in this 44-year-old epileptic woman.

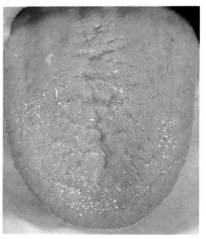

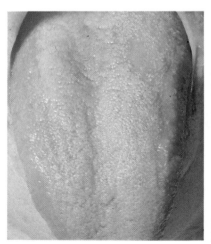

99

100

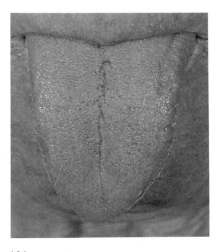

101 Mildly coated tongue of an elderly female recovering from acute urinary tract infection. She was only able to take fluids over the previous 3 days.

102 A coated tongue associated with bronchopneumonia giving cyanosis in an 84-year-old woman sent to hospital with a mild left-sided stroke.

103 A large heavily coated tongue in a mildy depressed hypothyroid elderly male not eating because of depression.

101

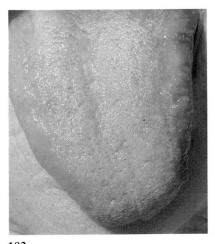

102

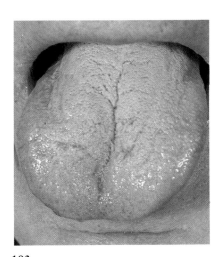

103

99 A mildly coated large tongue in a depressed older woman with reduced haemoglobin levels on blood test. Pallor definitely suggests a need for investigation of the folate deficiency anaemia. The large size would also justify investigation for hypothyroidism.

100 74-year-old woman admitted to hospital after 3 days of not eating. X-ray shows symptomless extensive pneumonia. Note definite cyanosis and anaemia.

104 Coated tongue from 72-year-old woman attending day-patient programme for arthritis. Note mild atrophy at the tongue edges. Polypharmacy (she was on six drugs including phenothiazine which may have been responsible) is a possible cause of brown pigmentation – unexplained as she is a non-smoker.

105 75-year-old Maori, retired army officer, with a heavy coating of the tongue, probably related to loss of dentures.

106 Heavily coated atrophic tongue in an elderly woman with atheromatous disease who was hospitalised for rehabilitation.

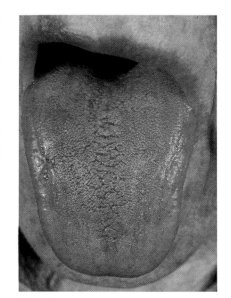

104

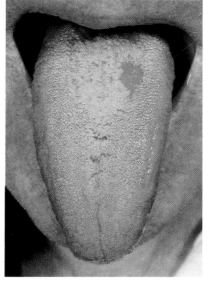

105

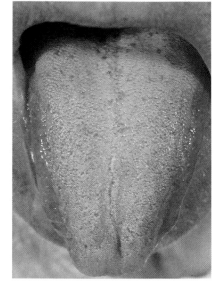

106

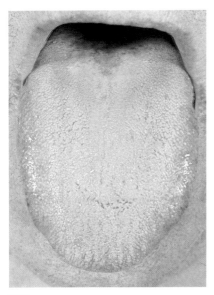

107

107 Large heavily coated tongue in a very old man with digoxin toxicity, congestive heart failure and depression. Some chromogenic bacterial over-growth, confirmed by swab analysis, probably related to sequential courses of tetracyclines and amoxycillin.

108 72-year-old day patient with mild renal failure, on drugs but non-smoker. Abnormal coating due to dietary factors and failure of immune mechanisms allowing coloration of the tongue from pathogenic bacteria and fungi.

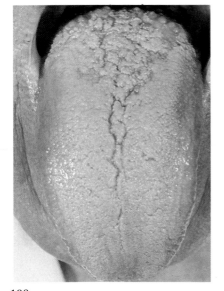

108

Table 3 Fur on the tongue
(Filiform papillae hypertrophy)

Increases
    Smokers
    Fasting
    Poorly fitting or absent dentures
    Dentures not used for eating
    Soft processed food diets

Decreases
    Vegetarians
    High fibre diets
    Broad spectrum antibiotics
    Habitual toothbrushing of tongue

109 Heavy coating of tongue in an elderly hermit with no teeth. The coating emphasises the structure of the root of the tongue and hides the nutritional glossitis.

110 Mild 'fur' in emphysematous old man who continues to smoke surreptitiously. Note fur in deep central fissure and mild cyanosis, secondary to lung disease.

111 Elderly retired widower. Pipe smoking gives marked central and posterior 'fur'.

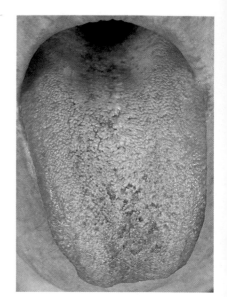

109

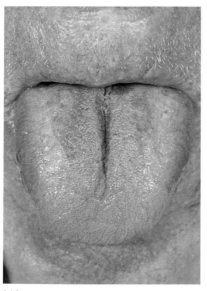

110

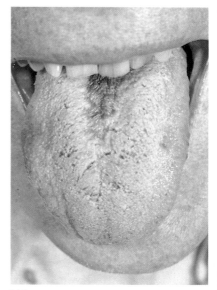

111

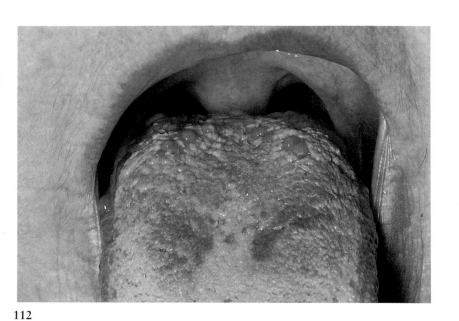

112

112 Dark candidal 'fur' confined to middle third of tongue in a middle-aged woman.

113 Extreme filiform hypertrophy of the mid and posterior tongue in a debilitated cancer patient with a changed microbial growth.

114 Close-up of middle third of the tongue of a 63-year-old male with 'hairy' tongue (brown fur) well demonstrated.

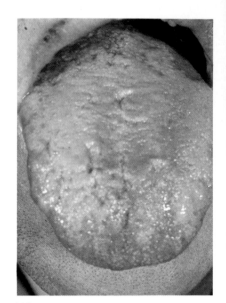

113

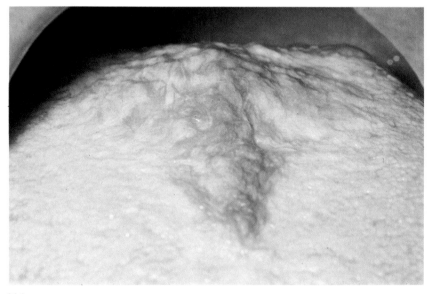

114

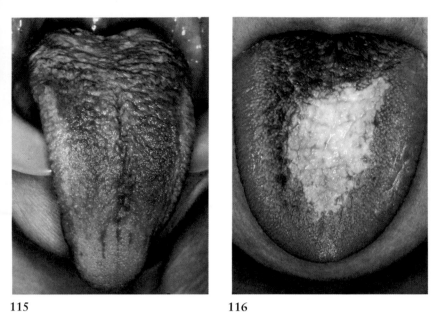

115   **116**

115 Extreme example of black hairy tongue in a Glaswegian.

116 A 'black and white' tongue. Some leukoplakia in the front third of a black hairy tongue.

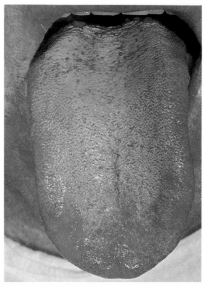 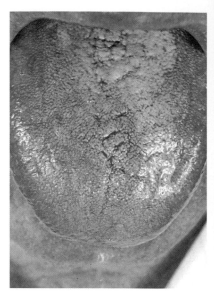

117   118

117 and 118 The coating on the tongue may be clean on one edge where more movement occurs. This can be seen in these two elderly patients with unilateral pyramidal tract signs but with no limb weakness present.

119 Good example of half-cleaned coating on the tongue. The hemiparetic or weak side also shows early tongue wasting but no deviation to the side of the lesion.

120 Unusual tongue coating in plethoric 58-year-old woman with hypertrophic pulmonary arthropathy.

121-123 Coatings of the tongue are commonly bacterial or monilial. *Candida albicans* or 'thrush' can give a variety of appearances ranging from diffuse coatings to patchy lesions. More rarely, plaques may replace a general coating of *Candida*.

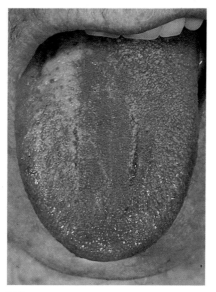

119

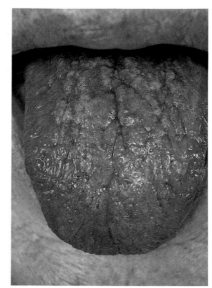

120

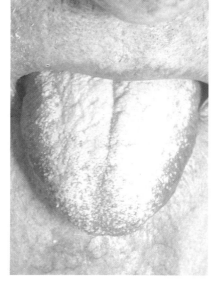

121

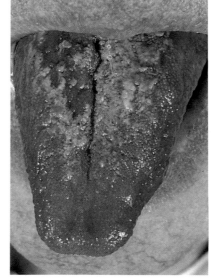

122

85

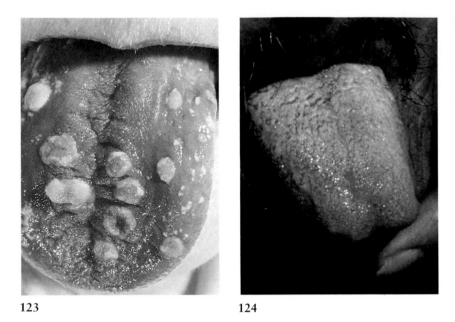

123   124

124 In this man from the Indian sub-continent, the coated tongue appears enlarged because of the loss of the teeth.

References

Beaven D.W., Easton B.H., (Eds). Changing ideas of disease, evolution for survival. In: *The Future of New Zealand Medicine* N.M. Peryer Limited, Christchurch, New Zealand, 1974, pp7-11.

Bomford R., Mason S., Swash M. *Hutchison's Clinical Methods*, 16th edn. Bailliere Tindall, London, 1975, pp39-40.

McCarthy P.L., Shklar G. *Diseases of the Oral Mucosa*, 2nd edn. Lea and Febiger, Philadelphia, 1980, pp4-17.

McLeod J., Munro J. *Clinical Examination*, 7th edn, Churchill Livingstone, Edinburgh, 1986, p76.

Chapter 7

'Portcullis' Syndrome and Angular Stomatitis

Elderly patients with slowly shrinking alveolar ridges may have had dentures or dental plates moulded many years previously. A growing mismatch can occur between the rigid and fixed dentures and the absorbing and changing gum shape. Not only does the hard dental material rub small ulcers, but suction of the upper dentures is increasingly lost. When the elderly patient, sitting up in bed, 'drops off' to sleep, the lower jaw often falls open.

In some patients, loose upper dentures may fall down, like a portcullis 'guarding the open mouth'. Portcullis syndrome is a condition when the upper teeth fall to protect the open mouth during sleep (Anonymous, 1986). It is highly relevant that loose dentures cause micro and mini-ulcers which produce pain when acidic foods are eaten. Older people with loose dentures thus avoid acidic foods, including ascorbic acid or Vitamin C.

In a series of 70 men more than 75 years of age, scurvy and Vitamin B deficiency were found to correlate with loose or ill-fitting dentures (Beaven, 1976). At this time as other B vitamin levels could not be measured but thiamin plasma and red cell levels were available these were taken as a general measure of B deficiency. The gum and alveolar ridge shrinkage continues and unless the dentures are constantly remoulded outwards, the corners of the mouth also fall inwards. Saliva can more easily run from the angle of the lips, producing cracks at the corners of the mouth. Angular stomatitis, or cracks on the lips or cheilitis is thus also significantly more common in the elderly with loose fitting dentures who also more often have nutritional deficiencies. Angular stomatitis, Portcullis syndrome and a heavily coated tongue in febrile elderly patients will alert the astute general clinical observer or health worker to nutritional deficiency states. These can be confirmed by blood screens and plasma nutritional indices, together with leucocyte Vitamin C or plasma B vitamin levels (McClean, 1976 a & b). It should be emphasised that the findings of such loose dentures by the primary health care worker implies a mandatory referral to a qualified dentist.

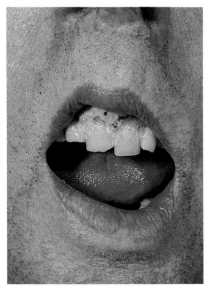 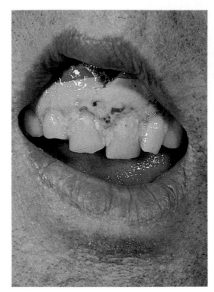

125   126

125-129 A good example of the 'portcullis syndrome' in an elderly European male with recent weight loss and poorly-fitting, out-dated 30-year-old dentures which have not been relined. These are dropping to guard the entrance to his mouth as he goes to sleep, and the lower jaw opens. Such loose dentures and 'portcullis syndrome' are invariably associated with nutritional deficiencies just visible in glossitis, at the tongue tip in **125** and **126**.

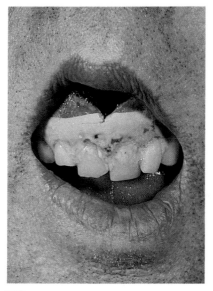

127

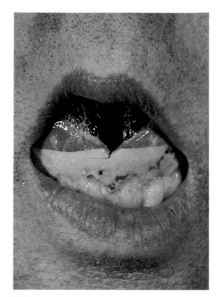

128

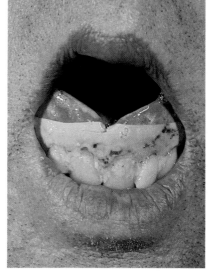

129

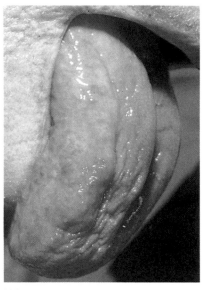

130

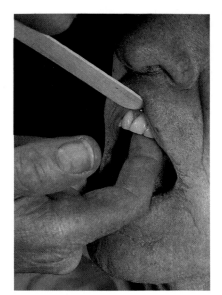

131

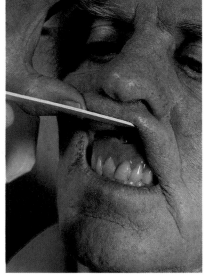

132

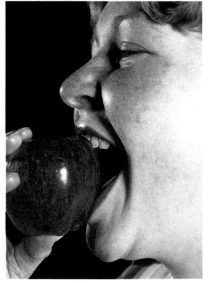

133

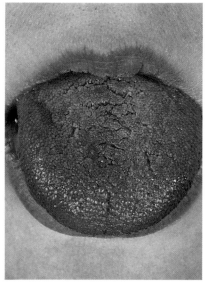

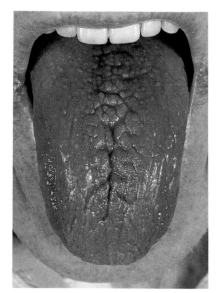

134   135

130 The tongue from an elderly female with 'portcullis syndrome' where atrophy of filiform papillae dominates the clinical picture, giving rise to a smooth pale tongue and iron deficiency anaemia.

131 Where glossitis is present and suspected to be of nutritional origin, the 'fit' of dentures should be examined. Before referring to the dentist, the non-dental health worker can identify the 'fit' and suction of the upper dental plate by pulling down with the forefinger.

132 Loosely fitting dentures are demonstrated in this elderly man.

133 An example of the way in which healthy teeth and gums allow an apple to be sharply bitten into.

134 Angular stomatitis related to dietary changes in a young woman. Angular stomatitis has resulted from her lack of nutritional knowledge and documented poor selection of vitamin containing foods, rather than inadequate dental apparatus.

135 'Portcullis syndrome' with nutritional changes. Angular stomatitis or cheilitis is present at the corners of the mouth. Note the deep central fissure in the tongue. It should be noted that it is the lack of vertical dimension in ageing dentures which has predisposed to these changes.

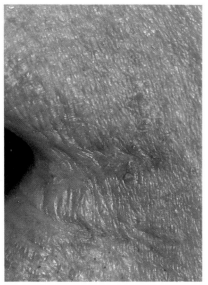 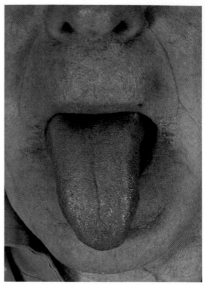

136   **137**

136   Angular lesions at the corner of the mouth in an edentulous old woman.

137   Widespread angular cracks due to saliva flow, secondary to worn dentures, which have a lack of vertical dimension.

References

Anonymous. Portcullis syndrome terminology developed because of the widespread use of such 'loose and ill-fitting dentures'. Undergraduate teaching texts in Christchurch, New Zealand from the 1960s.

Beaven D.W. Diet, dentistry and disease. *NZ Dental J* 1976, **72**, 68-74.

McClean H.E. *et al.* Nutrition of elderly men living alone. Vitamin C and Thiamine status. *NZ J Med* 1976, **84**, 345-48.

McClean H.E. *et al.* Nutrition of elderly men living alone. Intakes of energy and nutrients. *NZ Med J* 1976, **84**, 305-309.

Chapter 8
Ulcers of the Tongue

An excellent review on this topic starts with 'Most mouth ulcers are caused by *trauma* or are *aphthous*' (Grattan & Scully, 1986).

However, with the widespread use of pharmacological drugs in increasing numbers of older patients, what starts as a low-grade chronic glossitis can progress to a small visible ulcer. Some ulcers may occur in patients with connective tissue diseases and autoimmune disorders such as Sjögren's syndrome (Mason *et al.*, 1973) or Behçet's syndrome (Yazici *et al.*, 1984). Patients with rheumatoid arthritis are usually on a variety of drugs. It should be emphasized that non-steroidal drugs can be a potent and frequent cause of direct ulceration.

Sjögren's syndrome is typified by a reduction in the flow of tears and saliva. Thus a 'sicca' syndrome or dry mouth results which is much more susceptible to minor trauma. In this condition papillary atrophy may masquerade as superficial ulceration. In Behçet's syndrome, recurrent aphthous ulceration occurs in association with genital ulceration and uveitis. Cummings (1973) describes the mouth and tongue ulcerations seen in an extensive variety of connective tissue diseases.

Traumatic ulcers can sometimes be sorted out by careful examination of contact points in a good light, although we have seen persistent ulceration where a metal or amalgam 'filling' in a tooth has been persistently sharpened.

Recurrent aphthous ulcers, also sometimes called aphthae or aphthous stomatitis, occur in all areas with the exception of the hard palate and gingivae. They can be seen on the top and under the tongue. They may be alone or in small groups and usually persist for 3-10 days. Their cause is not clear but some reviews suggest they are more common in nutritional deficiencies or secondary to diseases in the small gut. Minor aphthous ulcers appear to affect quite large numbers of teenagers and young adults in most of whom no pathological background can be found (Rennie *et al.*, 1985; Ferguson *et al.*, 1984).

However, ulceration due to more general skin disorders such as lichen planus or pemphigoid syndromes are often larger, more irregular and usually associated with quite severe desquamative gingivitis. Some mouth and tongue ulcers can occur in viral infections where associated clinical features will help in the diagnosis.

The recently described 'magic syndrome' has, as its main feature, mouth and genital ulcers with inflamed cartilage (Firenstein *et al.*, 1985) somewhat similar to Behçet's syndrome.

Ulcerations in the tongue edges can be part of general medical disorders or specific gut disease (Cooke *et al.*, 1977; Borroni *et al*, 1984). The ulceration seen in association with neutropenia from drugs or radical oncology treatment programmes are, as in infectious mononucleosis, found more in the lymphoid tissue at the root of the tongue (Gayford & Haskell, 1979).

In some patients, Reiter's disease and sexually transmitted diseases such as HIV infections as well as gonococcal and syphilitic disorders, can give mouth ulcers, sometimes occurring on the tongue.

Lastly, in appropriate age groups, chronic ulceration always raised the possibility of malignancy, often only resolved by biopsy (McCarthy & Shklar, 1980). Tongue ulcers share much of the pathological background of other oral ulceration but patients usually expect careful and close examination of the tongue. Any tongue ulcer needs to be investigated in the context of age, history, including drug history and general skin or connective tissue disorder before referring for an opinion from an oral medicine specialist who may feel a biopsy is required.

Table 4 Major causes of tongue ulceration

Recurrent aphthous
Glossitis from drugs and nutritional disorders
Dental and electrolytic
Rheumatic diseases and Behçet's syndrome
Agranulocytosis and neutropenia
Reiter's and sexually transmitted diseases
Malignant ulcers
Systemic histoplasmosis granuloma with tongue ulceration

---

138 Aphthous ulcer of the tongue in otherwise healthy young woman.

139 Small visible aphthous ulcer of unknown origin near edge of tongue tip.

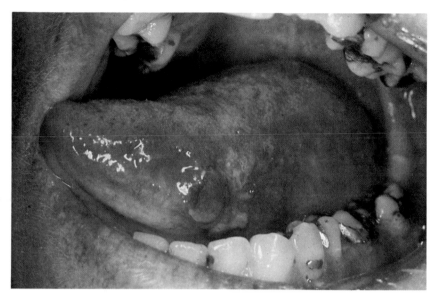

138

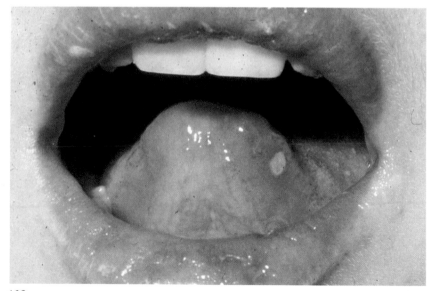

139

95

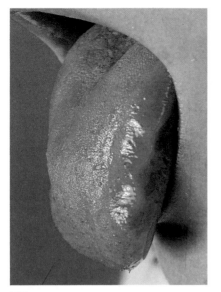

140

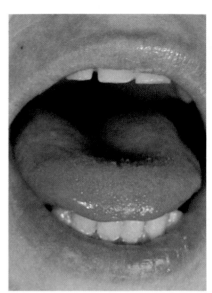

141

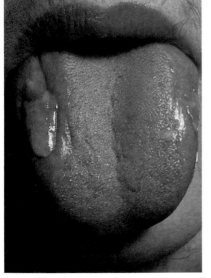

142

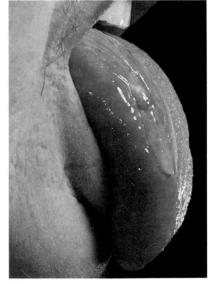

143

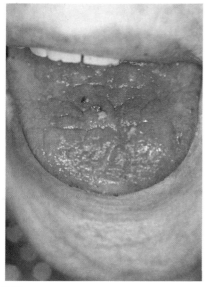

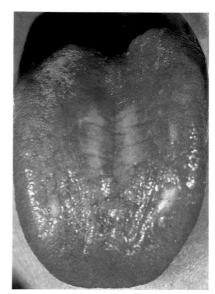

144   145

140   Several small aphthous ulcers on the left lateral edge of the tongue of a student nurse.

141   Three healing aphthous ulcers on the lower lip and one on left side of the tongue just visible in a teenage college student.

142 and 143   Very large superficial ulcer in a 65-year-old woman on anti-inflammatory drugs. An area of breaking-down glossitis.

144   Small ulcer with some pigmentation in 70-year-old woman with Behçet's disease.

145   Very superficial small ulcer near base of tongue on the left side in association with to Sjögren's syndrome.

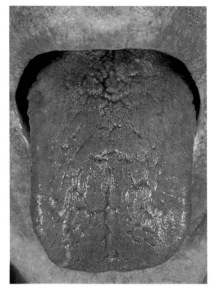

146

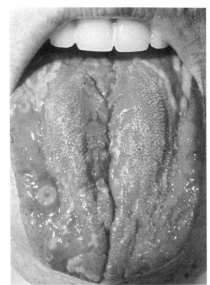

147

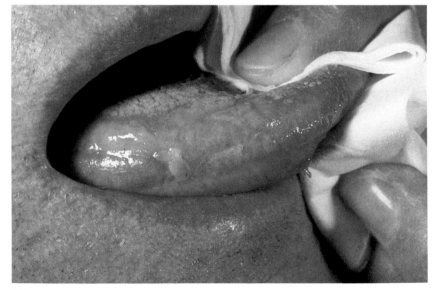

148

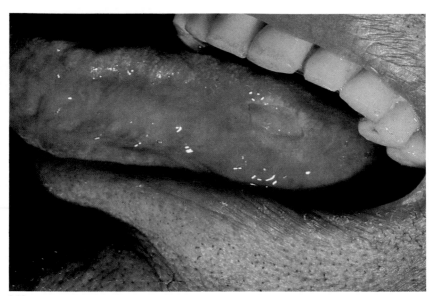

149

146 71-year-old woman with a painful red tongue. Indomethacin-induced glossitis has led to a small superficial ulcer near the right posterior edge.

147 84-year-old man with coronary heart disease and emphysema showing mild cyanosis, and some posterior geographic tongue. There is a small superficial ulcer on the right anterior third of the tongue.

148 Small slough in an ulcer produced by sharp edge to an amalgam filling on the posterior edge (R) of the tongue.

149 An ulcer (non-malignant by later biopsy) near posterior third on the ventral surface, probably caused by a very sharp isolated tooth spicule.

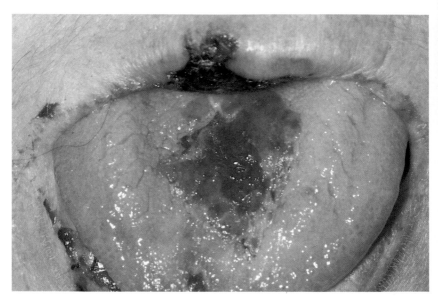

150

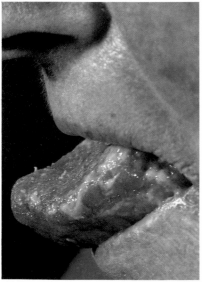

151

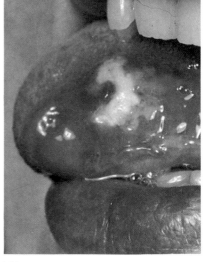

152

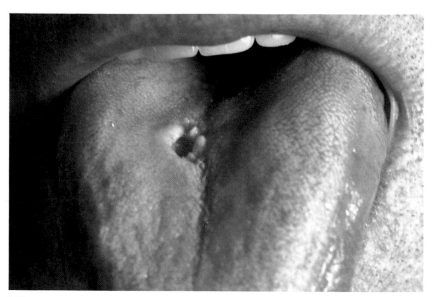

153

150 Debilitated old woman with chronic lymphatic leukaemia and large shadow ulcer on the dorsum of the tongue. Note that the ulcer is filled with debris and could be pemphigoid.

151 Ulcerated area on the left posterior edge of tongue in an older chronically ill woman. Note also dorsal tongue erosions.

152 Ulcer near the tip secondary to a tongue bite during a Grand Mal convulsion.

153 54-year-old accountant with some arthritis and an ulcer initially thought to be malignant. Biopsy showed this to be benign. Aetiology uncertain.

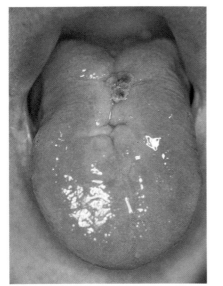

154

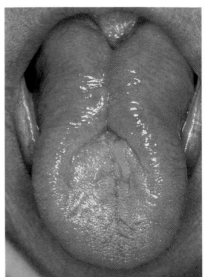

155

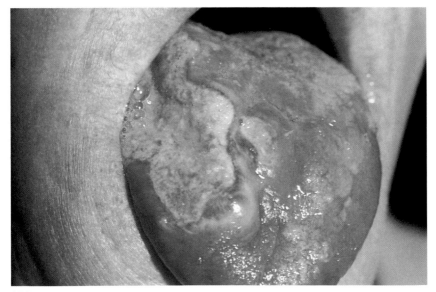

156

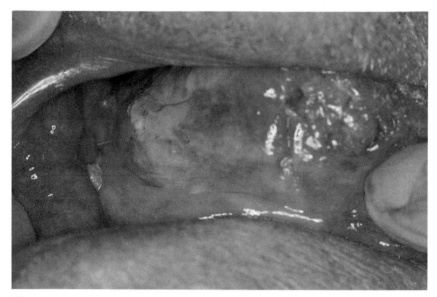

157

154 Elderly female smoker with pigmented ulcer and marked atrophic candidiasis (previous antibiotic treatment) of the tongue. Biopsy revealed a squamous cell cancer.

155 After resection of a part of the centre of the tongue and repair.

156 Extensive superficial ulceration typical of cancer of the tongue which was confirmed in the cytology from biopsy.

157 Painful posterior edge of the right side of the tongue, superficial ulceration and an indurated area of squamous cell cancer.

References

Borroni G., Pericoli R., Gabba P. *et al*. Eosinophilic ulcers of the tongue. *J Cutan Pathol* 1984, **11**(4), 322-325.

Cooke B.E.D., Challacombe S., Rose M.S., *et al*. Recurrent oral ulceration. *Proc Roy Soc Med* 1977, **70**, 354-357.

Cummings N.A. The oral mucosal manifestations of rheumatic diseases In: *Rheumatology: An Annual Review*. Karger, Basle, 1973, pp60-97.

Firenstein G.S., Gruber H.E., Weisman M.H. *et al*. Mouth and genital ulcers with inflamed cartilage: Magic Syndrome. *Amer J Med* 1985, **79**, 65-71.

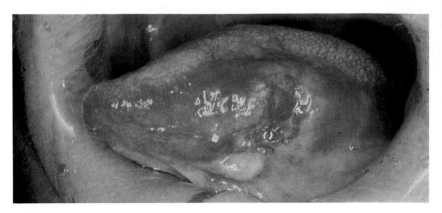

158

158 61-year-old woman, heavy smoker, showing ulcer due to squamous cell carcinoma of the tongue, extending into the floor of the mouth and proving unresponsive to radiotherapy. Later, a hemiglossectomy was carried out.

Ferguson M.M. Carter J., Boyle P. An epidemiological study of factors associated with recurrent aphthae in women. *J Oral Med* 1984, **39**, 212.

Gayford J.J., Haskell R. *Clinical Oral Medicine*, 2nd edn. John Wright, Bristol, 1979, pp1-17.

Grattan C.E.H., Scully C. Oral ulceration: A diagnostic problem. *Br Med J* 1986, **292**, 1093-1094.

Hindle M.O., Franklin C.D. Food allergy on intolerance in severe recurrent aphthous ulceration of the mouth. *Br Med J* 1986, **292**, 1237-1238.

Mason A.M.S., Gumpel J.M., Golding P.L. Sjögren's syndrome – a clinical review. *Seminars in Arthritis and Rheumatism* 1973, **II**(4), 301-331.

McCarthy P.L., Shklar G. *Diseases of the Oral Mucosa*. 2nd edn. Lea & Febiger, Philadelphia, 1980, pp132-136, 407 & 408, 471 & 472.

Rennie J.S., Reade P.C., Hay K.D. *et al*. Recurrent aphthous stomatitis. *Br Dent J* 1985, **159**, 361-367.

Yazici H., Chamberlain M.A., Tuzun Y. *et al*. A comparative study of pathergy reaction among Turkish and British patients with Behçet's disease. *Ann Rheum Dis* 1984, **43**, 74-75.

Chapter 9
Acute Glossitis, Including Drug-induced Glossitis

Any of the four types of papillae on the tongue can develop an acute inflammatory response with shedding of surface epithelium. The most commonly affected are the most numerous tall filiform papillae with their immensely fast turnover of the superficial cells. Thus any chemical substances which reach the surface epithelium by means of the saliva or the rich blood supply, may affect the daily turnover of cells on the filiform papillae (McCarthy & Shklar, 1980). Systemic drugs may affect the tongue as part of a true allergy in the oral cavity or gut as a whole, or purely as an idiosyncratic reaction.

Thus a drug's side-effect, or general reaction may involve the oral mucous membrane or the gingiva but not the tongue. In other patients, some oral or mucous membrane reaction is found as well as skin changes and, sometimes, a dry mouth and dry tongue with mild glossitis are the only reactions. The glossitis and painful tongue which may be the chief complaint may be associated with other physical signs such as pursing of the lips, protrusion of the tongue and mouth, smacking movements and even trismus. Associated rashes, arthralgias or other general medical signs or symptoms may assist in these differential diagnoses of which several drugs are responsible (Dreisen, 1984).

The areas between the filiform papillae may also accumulate toxic chemical substances. Because of the very high rate of cell replication on the filiform papillae, they are also especially sensitive to minor deficiencies in nutrients. Thus, early signs of micronutrient substance deficiencies such as iron and vitamins may be seen first in mild glossitis. If more severe, then the nerve endings for pain are more superficial, giving rise to a burning sensation over the tip and even over the main dorsum of the tongue (Cawson, 1969).

Many of the antibiotics which, with time, can produce an acute atrophic candidiasis act by both altering bacterial flora in the mouth and also by acting on the small gut to reduce absorption of specific nutrients and vitamins. Because the surface epithelium gradually becomes thinner with age, older patients have significantly reduced numbers of epithelial cells. In addition, drug clearance is reduced, thus making them particularly prone to acute drug-induced glossitis. A controversial study of a defined population in Sweden was carried out by Axell in 1976.

Since that time, it is possible that drug-induced glossitis in older patients has become more common, as various forms of acute glossitis have appeared much more frequently in greater numbers of older hospitalised patients over the last decade. The most common causes of glossitis are infections or allergies in the young and nutritional or drug-induced states in the elderly.

Table 5 Drugs affecting the tongue*

Analgesics	Phenylbutazone	+++
	Oxyphenbutazone	+++
	Naproxen	+
	Indomethacin	+
Antihypertensives	Methyldopa	++
Antibiotics	Tetracyclines (all)	++++
	Gentamicins and related aminoglycosides†	+
Cephalosporins	Chloramphenicol	++
	Anti-TB drugs	+
Antineoplastics	All	++
Heavy metals	High concentrations of gold, lead, bismuth, arsenicals, mercury	
Antispasmodics	i.e. Carbamazepine	
Antimalarials Penicillamine	i.e. Pyrimethamine	

* Observers should be aware that there is a widely differing range of drugs with different actions and different side-effects which may affect the tongue. Tongue symptoms or signs, caused by these drugs, may be better evaluated by referral to an oral medicine specialist.

† Related aminoglycosides: tobramycin; metelmycin; kanamycin; neomycin; amikacin; etc.

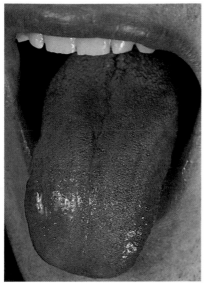 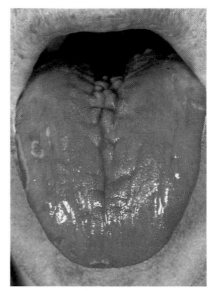

159   160

159 Acute allergic reaction to methocarbamol with painful edges to the tongue in a man who also has some hay fever and asthma.

160 Sub-acute glossitis in an older woman with painful tongue and loss of filiform papillae. Not related to drugs. Geographic tongue on right side of the tongue and at the tip.

Table 6 Major groupings of glossitis

Infections: bacterial, fungal or viral

Allergic and toxic and secondary to systemic disorders

Drug-induced (see major drug groups)

Nutritional: vitamin B12
            iron
            folic acid
            other B vitamins: niacin
                              riboflavin
                              pyridoxine

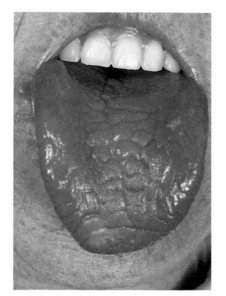

161

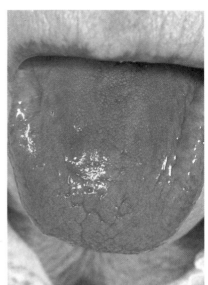

162

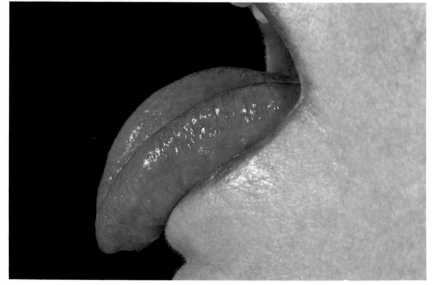

163

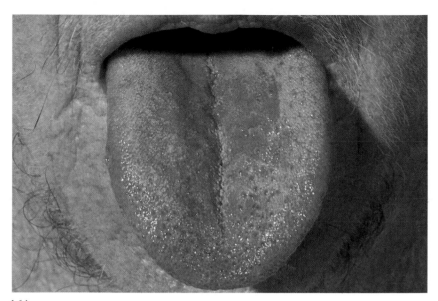

164

161 Acute response seen in an elderly woman after antimitotic drugs given for cancer therapy had ceased.

162 Chronic atrophic glossitis with associated widespread gastric atrophy. All the evidence is that such an association is secondary (both tongue surface and gastric mucosa arise from same primitive or endodermal foregut tissues).

163 Mild glossitis with painful edges to the tongue in a young woman athlete taking non-steroidal anti-inflammatory drugs.

164 Older woman with patchy diffuse glossitis, possibly due to repetitive use of phenol mouthwash.

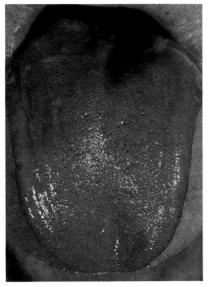

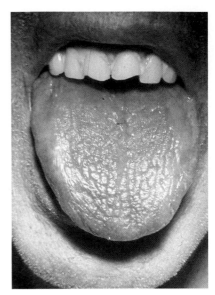

165 **166**

165 Acute atrophic candidiasis in elderly male given multiple courses of amoxycillin antibiotics.

166 Sub-acute superficial glossitis with smooth left edge to the tongue in a middle-aged Madrassi woman, cause unknown but possibly due, from the history, to food additives such as paprika, pepper and curry.

167 Very mild glossitis of the tip of the tongue only, in a 58-year-old male invalid smoking heavily and on carbamazepine and phenobarbitone. Dorsum of tongue shows possibly drug-induced glossitis only at the tip. Also pseudo-papillomatous cobble-stones at the right border. Heavy "smokers' fur" posteriorly.

168 22-year-old woman with behavioural disorder showing acute glossitis and dry mouth secondary to medication. Mild and local hyperplastic gingivitis of some kind likely to be secondary to the medical condition – probably poorly maintained oral hygiene. Medications: haloperidol, benzotropine mesylate, bromide mixtures and methotrimeprazine.

169 85-year-old outpatient attending rehabilitation after cancer chemotherapy with vinblastine and adriamycin.

170 Acute drug-induced glossitis in a 55-year-old single Polynesian male slaughter-man. Superficial erosions and swelling of the tongue with previous thick coating still remaining. History of high alcohol intake suggests previous nutritional deficiencies plus drug allergy. Anti-inflammatory medication with ketoprofen in high dosage and methyldopa were being taken. Improved when drugs were discontinued.

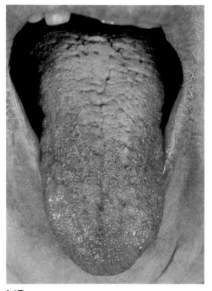

167

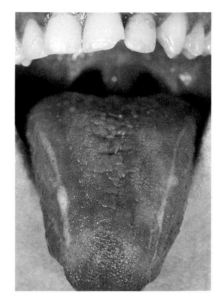

168

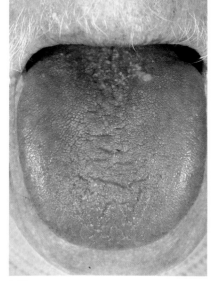

169

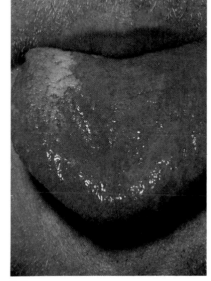

170

111

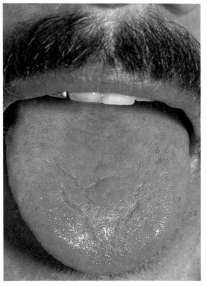 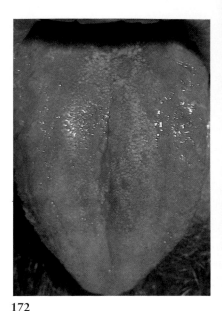

171 172

171 Very mild superficial glossitis in Malaysian labourer recently treated with unusually high-dose amoxycillin therapy for resistant lung infection.

172 Acute glossitis in a young 29-year-old farmer inappropriately treated with tetracyclines for Coxsackie B virus infection.

173 97-year-old lady lapsed in her attendances for Vitamin B12 injections for 20 years' pernicious anaemia. She also has marked gastric atrophy and antibodies documented.

174 Lilac-coloured atrophic tongue in old woman presenting with heart failure secondary to gross iron deficiency anaemia. Koilonychia was also marked in the finger and toenails.

175 Some nutritional glossitis and mild anaemia in elderly lonely widower thought to be depressed and not eating.

176 Early atrophic glossitis with mild pernicious anaemia.

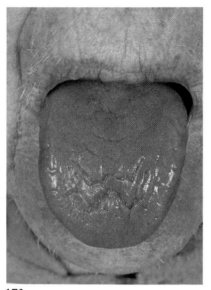

173

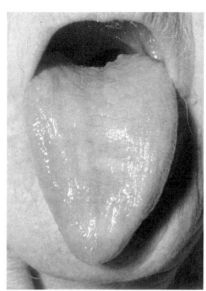

174

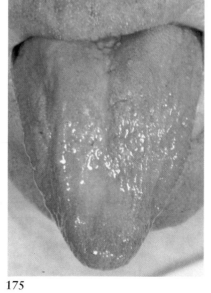

175

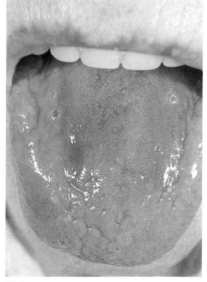

176

177 Chronic atrophic glossitis with iron and folate deficiency. Some early left heart failure has led to a bluish tinge to the tongue.

178 Tongue of chronic alcoholic. Multiple B deficiencies with reduced B12, riboflavin and thiamine levels.

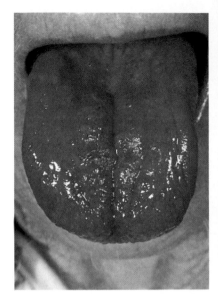

177

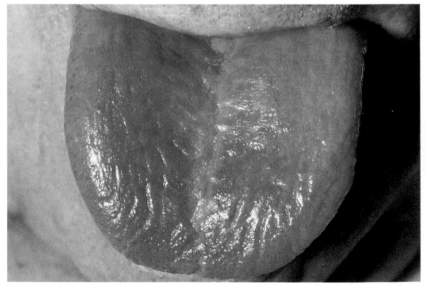

178

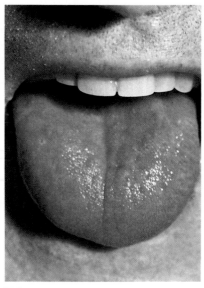 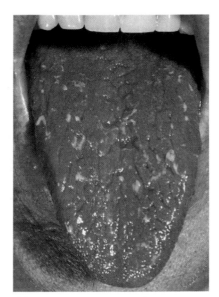

179   180

179   Middle-aged alcoholic barman with sub-acute glossitis from severe nutritional deficiences, including multiple B deficiency.

180   Elderly alcoholic pensioner with beri beri blood levels of thiamine. Chronic atrophic glossitis secondary to associated B vitamin deficiencies and flecks of thrush – possibly with some associated atrophic areas.

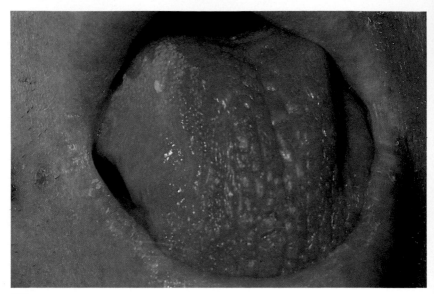

181

181 Strawberry-red glossitis in young male with radiation damage to the small gut and subsequent severe anorexia. Area of thrush extending on right side of tongue. Probably combined drug-induced glossitis also present from multiple medication.

References

Axell T. A prevalence study of oral mucosal lesions in an adult Swedish population. *Odontol Rev* 1976, **27**, Suppl 36.

Cawson R.A. Sore tongue. *Br J Dermatol* 1969, **81**, 462-463.

Dreisen S. Systemic significance of glossitis decoding the tongue's medical messages. *Postgrad Med* 1984, **75**, 207-215.

McCarthy P.L., Shklar G. *Diseases of the Oral Mucosa*. 2nd edn. Lea & Febiger, Philadelphia, 1980, pp35-58.

Chapter 10
Geographic Tongue or Glossitis Areata Migrans

In the past other terms have been used to describe this loss of filiform papillae in well-defined areas which become surrounded by a white edge representing disordered and possibly regenerating papillae. Because of the loss of papillae and hyperaemia, the geographic areas can vary between bright red and pale pink, but often have a piled-up or elevated white edge. A *map-like* appearance of the tongue results. Especially is this so as the lesions tend to migrate forward on the tongue. Some writers describe a microscopic appearance of pustules with later exfoliation and exposure of flattened papillae. Healing can slowly follow over days or weeks, but the lesions may resolve more slowly over months or years. In some cases lesions may persist for some years. A review by Hume (1975) sets out clearly that 1-2% of the population at any time may be affected, with a frequency of up to 15% in Jewish and Japanese children. This critical review of existing literature suggests that there is no sex or racial difference (except in Jewish children), that children are more commonly affected, and that the lesions of geographia occur more commonly in those tongues with more marked fissures.

Parakeratosis, acanthosis and permanent thinning of the epithelium of some papillae, seen in both this condition and the rare psoriasis of the tongue, suggest these disorders may be non-specific reactions to unknown factors.

Although geographic tongue has been reported to be more common in connective tissue disorders and rheumatoid arthritis, critical comparative studies for this association are lacking. There does appear to be an association with:

past history of hayfever, eczema or asthma;
family history of geographic tongue;
family history of hayfever, eczema or asthma;
raised levels of immunoglobulin E < 200 units/ml.

In a comparison (Robin & Simons, 1979) between 80 patients and 225 normals without geographic tongue, there appeared to be an increased incidence of reaction to five common allergens (house dust mite, rye grass pollen, cat epithelial material, air-borne moulds and whole cows' milk). But geographic tongue can persist for years in normal healthy subjects or it can develop fairly acutely in association with Reiter's disease, pustular psoriasis

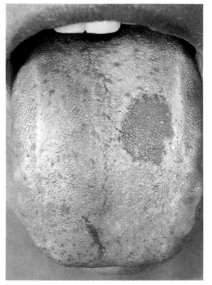

182

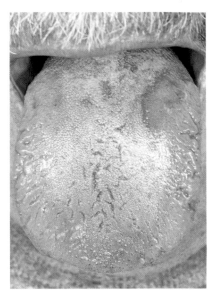

183

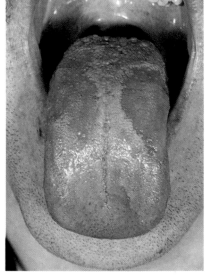

184

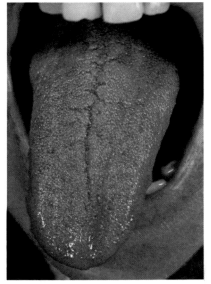

185

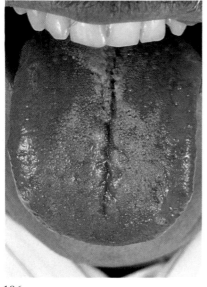
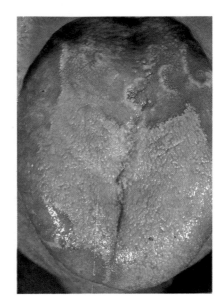

186 187

182 Normal healthy young physician with Type I migratory geographic lesions of the usual type.

183 62-year-old lawyer in good health though with one discrete patch and small areas of geographia. No known illness.

184 27-year-old male invalid with fixed geographic lesions and some mild athetosis not requiring medication. Circumvallate papillae seen.

185 Two small posterior lesions in a young man who has also been prescribed high doses of chlorpromazine.

186 Sixteen years of migratory geographic tongue in an ex-pipe-smoking 35-year-old doctor.

187 Widespread obvious lesions on the surface of an enlarged tongue from an elderly woman. Hypothyroidism was suggested as the cause of the enlarged tongue.

and in acute autoimmune disorders such as acute disseminated lupus erythematosis. No definite evidence for a genetic origin or for chromosome or genetic markers has been identified as yet (Correll *et al.*, 1984).

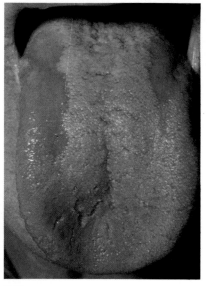

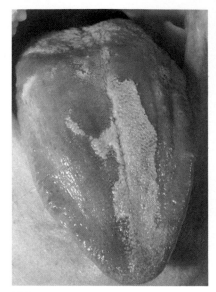

188   189

Table 7 Geographic stomatitis

Type I		Only on dorsum and sides of tongue. Migratory. Active and remission phases (usual picture)
Type II	**A**	Fixed forms or non-migratory (lingua geographia) occur and recur in the same place
	B	Yellowish-white patches occur and recur in the same areas but do not show full-blown redness of exfoliation
Type III		'Geographic' lesions on surfaces other than the tongue

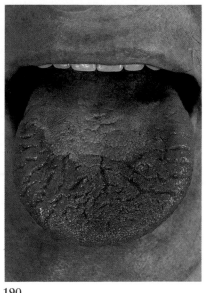

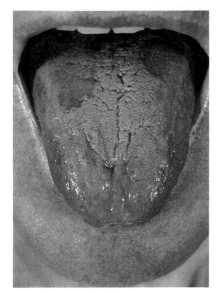

190

191

188 Geographic and migratory lesions for some years in a 50-year-old gardener. Coincidentally there is also a definite history of allergy to cats.

189 Small amounts of residual epithelium between the areas of mild glossitis form the geographic pattern in this elderly man of mixed Chinese ancestry.

190 Possible Type II geographic tongue with acute onset in an Italian shopkeeper. Some areas of atrophy on posterior gingiva.

191 Possible Type IIA lesions in an elderly pigmented male.

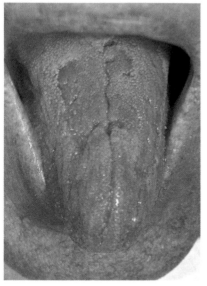 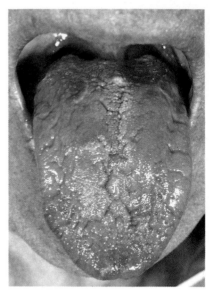

192

193

192 Young woman referred with Type IIIA lesions, but the history and lesion suggest probable Type I.

193 Elderly, retired male army officer with geographic lesions, probably Type IIB.

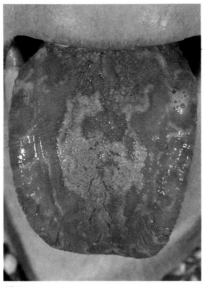 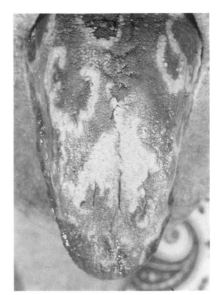

194 **195**

194 Older Indonesian man with obvious geographic tongue which could be classified as Type IIB.

195 Striking geographic pattern of a circular or annular type.

References

Correll R.W., Westcott W.B., Jensen J.L. Nonpainful erythematous circinate lesions of a protein nature on a fissured tongue. *J Amer Dent Assoc* 1984, **109**(1), 90-91.

Hume W.J. Geographic stomatitis. A critical review. *J Dentistry* 1975, 3(1), 25-43.

Robin M. Simons M.J. Geographic tongue – a manifestation of atopy. *Br J Derm* 1979, **101**, 159-162.

General Disorders with Clinical Signs on the Tongue

Any unusual changes in the dorsum of the tongue should prompt the curious clinical observer to ask the question: Are the appearances within the range of normality for age and sex? We have observed patients admitted unconscious to hospital whose previously bitten, and now healed, tongues suggested the diagnosis of Grand Mal convulsions. Likewise, injuries to children falling from bicycles and to young adult males in car accidents and on the sports field often leave quite major scars on the dorsum or the side of the tongue. Because of the major blood supply and the thick and rapidly renewing epithelium of the tongue, less severe tearing injuries heal well although substantial bleeding can occur at the time.

Different drug eruptions with a generalised response will often produce a swollen tongue – at its most acute in forms such as erythema multiforme with Stevens-Johnson syndrome where there is severe swelling of lips, gums and tongue with epithelial loss, all in association with skin eruptions of the multiforme type. It is said that continuous high levels in the plasma of phenytoin sodium may rarely produce a swollen or enlarged tongue as well as the more commonly recognised gum or gingival hyperplasia.

Blood disorders such as thombocytopenia with platelets below 20,000 may give spontaneous haemorrhages, and when bone marrow involvement from leukaemia and associated neoplasms is marked, acute haemorrhages can occur in the tongue. These may be seen separately or around areas of leukaemic infiltration. Likewise we have seen small haemorrhages in association with very low Vitamin C levels. Where no teeth remain the bleeding areas in scurvy may be particularly marked under the tongue as well as on the soft palate (Suyama *et al.*, 1982). Small haemorrhages on the uvula or soft palate assist greatly in the diagnosis of infectious mononucleosis, especially where ulceration is present in the tonsillar lymphoid tissues with exudate over the root of the tongue. Other less frequent bleeding disorders initially manifest themselves in the tongue with small, easily seen haemorrhages in the rapidly turning over epithelium (Nelson, 1973; Wood & Losowsky, 1982).

Fish bones, pieces of glass and other foreign bodies in food occasionally result in small 'torn' lesions on the dorsum or sides of the tongue. Arterial embolus or obstruction can also present with necrosis of part of the tongue (Allen, 1980; Siemssen *et al.*, 1985; Barfoed & Bretlau, 1984).

The many general medical disorders which give rise to changes in the colour of the tongue are dealt with separately. Muscle and specific wasting disease are also dealt with in Chapter 18. Some examples of the value of tongue appearances in clinical diagnosis are given in Table 8.

Table 8 General disorders with clinical signs on the tongue

Injuries
  Bitten tongues
  Sports injuries
  Injuries from Grand Mal convulsions
  Fishbones and foreign bodies

Disorders of blood and blood vessels
  Scurvy
  Leukaemias and lymphomas
  Bleeding disorders
  Telangiectasia

Side-effects from drugs and general systemic disorders
  Drug eruptions
  Sarcoid disease
  Cyanosis
  Diabetes
  Fungus infections

Involvement with gut disorders
  Crohn's disease
  Ulcerative colitis

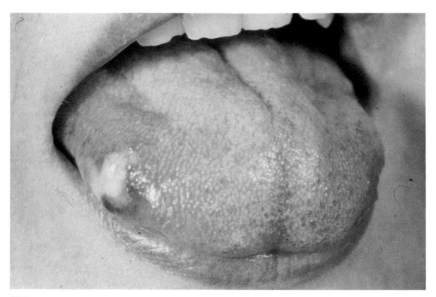

196

196 Acutely bitten tongue in a young woman with uncontrolled Grand Mal seizures.

197 Bitten tongue in a 60-year-old woman with generalised viral encephalitis and a fit. Note also "febrile" coated tongue.

198 Old scars in 45-year-old male epileptic secondary to teeth injury due to a fall during a fit. Some drug glossitis at edges of tongue. Medication: lorazepam, thioridazine hydrochloride, perphenazine and chlorpromazine hydrochloride.

199 Large scar from sporting injury in a young male with poor dietary habits.

200 Middle-aged alcoholic brewery worker with old injury to the tongue during a fall – almost certainly an alcoholic or 'rum' fit. Some nutritional glossitis.

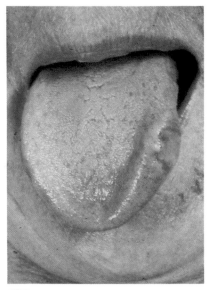

197

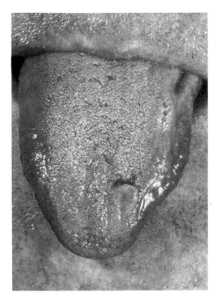

198

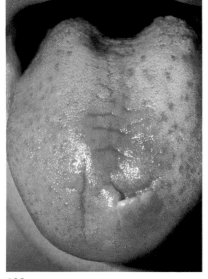

199

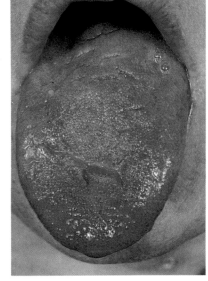

200

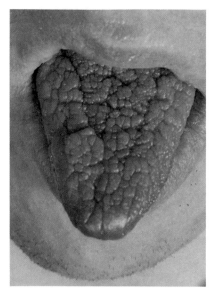

201

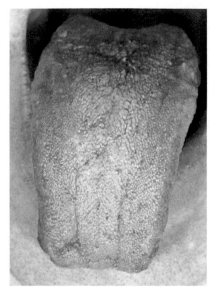

202

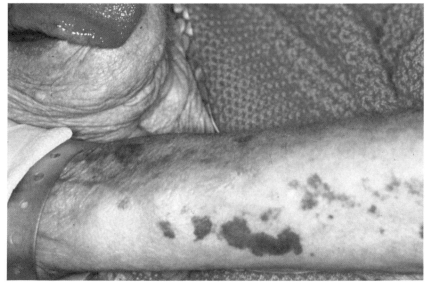

203

128

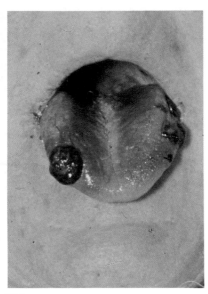

204

201 Young drug addict with marked scar on the right side of the tongue due to a previous fit. Note also some dehydration and glossitis.

202 46-year-old male with congenital mid-face underdevelopment. Unusual central or 'median rhomboid glossitis'. Small injury to right side of tongue tip, possibly due to theogotic damage from razor-sharp teeth.

203 Scurvy in an elderly female with gross nutritional changes and some microscopic haemorrhages in the tongue. Spontaneous bleeding was seen in the arms.

204 Presentation of spontaneous haemorrhages in the tongue of an elderly man with platelet count very low (below 12,000) possibly due to drug reaction.

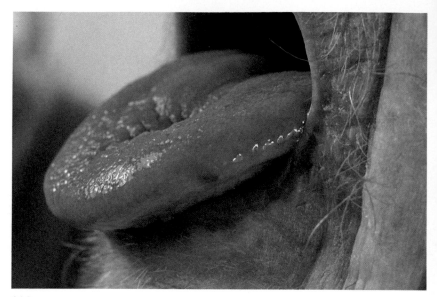

205

205 Venous telangiectasia with small venous loops.

206 Multiple hereditary familial telangiectasia on the tongue.

207 Multiple hereditary familial telangiectasia on the tip of the tongue and also on the lips.

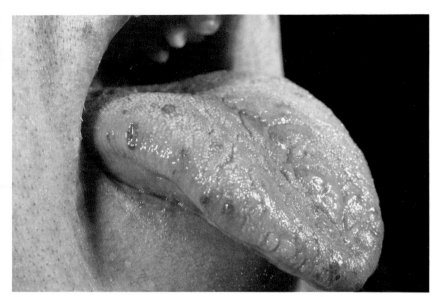

206

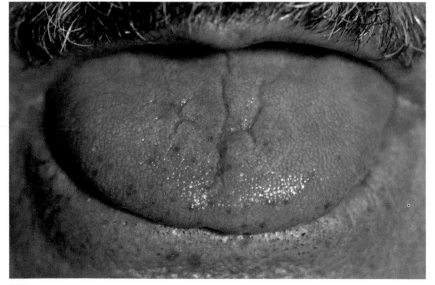

207

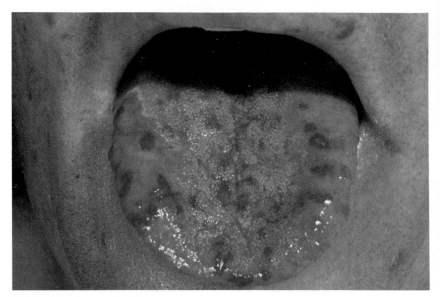

208

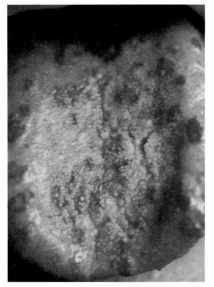

209

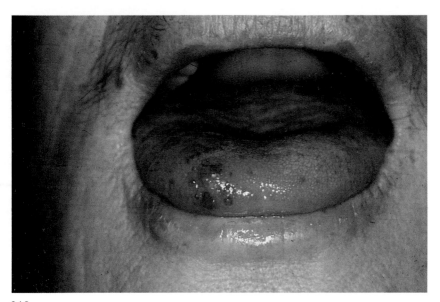

210

208 Very marked multiple hereditary telangiectasia of the tongue.

209 Relative of the patient shown in 208.

210 Hereditary telangiectasia (Osler type). Note also scattered small lesions on the lips.

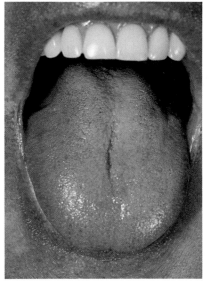

211

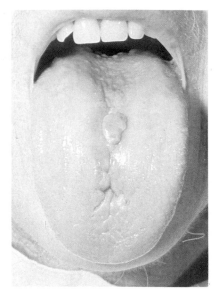

212

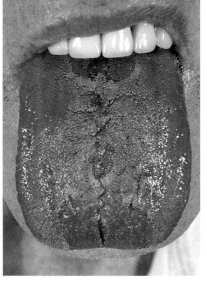

213

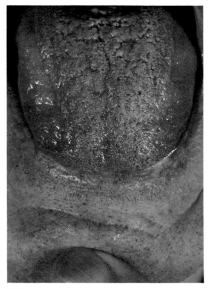

214

134

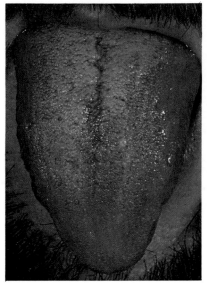
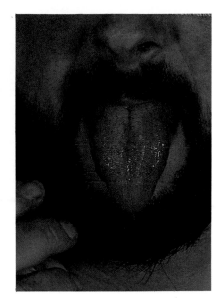

215   216

211 The rare syndrome of Peutz-Jeghers-Touraine with discrete pigmented patches (one on tongue) associated with gastrointestinal malignancy. Also usually seen on perioral skin and sometimes on the bridge of the nose. The syndrome is also associated with polyps of stomach and colon and the risk of carcinoma of the colon is great. Also linked to ovarian cancer.

212 Elderly woman with gross iron deficiency anaemia and a pale tongue.

213 Marked cyanosis of the face in a 74-year-old retired farmer showing a recent small stroke and oxygen desaturation. A large blue tongue and associated geographic tongue suggest the possibility of autoimmune hypothyroidism as the cause of this man's heart failure. Also suggested by low-voltage bedside ECG.

214 Tobacco-stained tongue and 'smoker's' finger.

215 and 216 Combined alcohol-nicotine-drug addiction in a young male with heavy smoking signs and coating on the tongue.

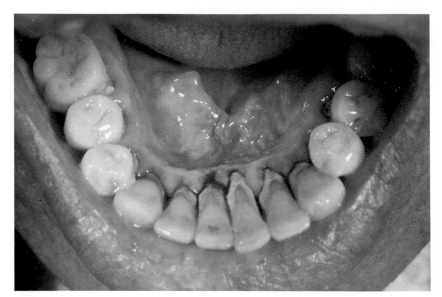

217

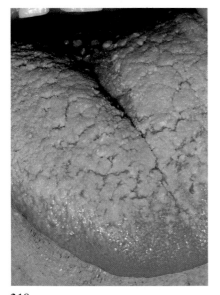

218

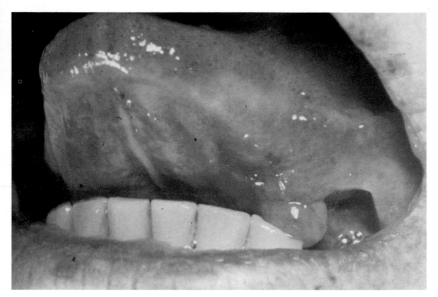

219

217 Lead poisoning in young Polynesian motor-car battery worker. Pigment under the tongue but more marked at the base of the teeth.

218 Candidial infection in a 52-year-old French chef presenting with previously undiagnosed diabetes mellitus or possibly HIV infections. Tenacious saliva and acetone on the breath may also suggest this diagnosis.

219 Crohn's disease of small gut with epithelial tag under the posterior tongue.

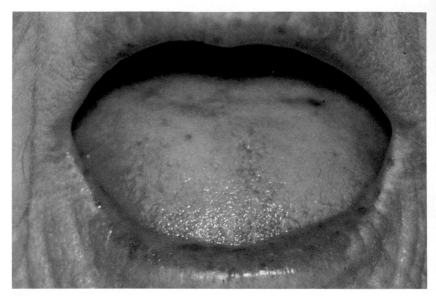

220

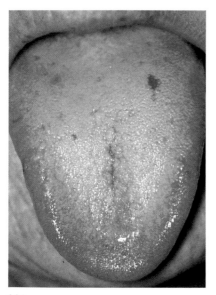

220 and 221 Systemic sclerosis in an elderly woman with characteristic narrowed and puckered mouth. The epithelium of the tongue is narrowed and atrophic with small blood vessels breaking through. Some sclerosis affects the small gut and there is associated mild jaundice. Scleroderma mainly affects skin (fingers, toes, perioral, thorax) and causes telangiectasis, oesophageal immotility, small bowel changes, malabsorption, diverticulosis coli, cardiac fibrosis, bundle branch blocks, pulmonary fibrosis with restrictive dysfunction, and a perfusion/diffusion impairment.

221

References

Allen P. Giant cell arteritis presenting with necrosis of the tongue – a case report. *Br J Oral Surg* 1980, **18**(2), 162-165.

Barfoed C.P., Bretlau P. Tongue necrosis in temporal arteritis. *Acta Otolaryngol* (Stockholm) 1984, **98**(3-4), 380-384.

Nelson H.C. Epidemic purpuric enanthem. *Irish Med Assn J* 1973, **66**(15), 507-511.

Siemssen S.J., Larsen O.D., McNair A. Necrotising tongue and skin lesions in temporal arteritis: Follow-up of a case with a possible iatrogenic factor. *Br Med J* 1985, **290**, 819-820.

Suyama H., Nakasono I., Yoshitake T., *et al*. Significance of haemorrhages in central parts of the tongue found in the medicolegal autopsy. *Forensic Sci Int* 1982, **20**(3), 256-258.

Wood G.M., Losowsky M.S. 'Angiodysplasia' of the tongue with acquired Von Willebrand's disease. *Postgrad Med J* 1982, **58**(675), 37-38.

Chapter 12

Vesiculo-bullous Diseases of the Tongue

With the tongue's thick and rapidly turning over surface layer of epithelial cells, it is not surprising that some disorders produce necrosis and fluid collection, either within the epithelium or between the epithelium and the lamina propria. Vesicles are small collections of fluid and bullae, caused by a split along the tissue layer, are the same pathological collections of fluid, but to a much larger degree caused by increased hydrostatic pressure or tension. Eventually the lesions break down to form ulcers.

Acute viral infections cause simple vesicular lesions, especially *Herpes simplex* and Coxsackie viruses.

Erythema multiforme is a more common disorder, often of younger patients, seen in response to many drug reactions or less common acute viral illnesses. This is a common condition. Cutaneous and sometimes mouth eruptions occur with swelling and vesicles. Some of these become confluent with widespread erosions affecting predominantly the lips although the tongue and mucous membrane can also be affected. The eroded areas heal with painful crusting. Other verruculo-bullous lesions may initially present as ulcerations (Lynch, 1984). In many cases no cause is found for the erythema multiforme. **Stevens-Johnson syndrome** is a more serious form with marked exudative features. Some patients present with gross swelling of lips and mouth. The surface of the tongue is also affected by the generalised inflammation.

Pemphigus vulgaris is a rare disorder. There are bullae around the mouth initially, later spreading to various areas of the skin. Abnormal epithelial cells seen in smears are called acantholytic cells. The bullae continue to spread, splitting and blistering off the skin. Without high-dose steroids and immuno-suppressants treatment the disorder, which appears to have an autoimmune basis and an increasingly high ESR, is fatal (Anderson & Kissane, 1984).

Pemphigoid is, in comparison, a benign and more common disease. There are two commonly-seen forms – the bullous pemphigoid and the less florid benign membrane mucosal variety (BMMP). The lesions usually start around the mouth and tongue and also affect the genitalia. They can also be seen as problems in the conjunctivae. Here the disorder is less florid, rarely affects the skin and runs a benign course. Unlike pemphigus, seen more often in 20 to 40-year-olds and more in females, pemphigoid is usually seen in patients in their sixties and seventies. Such patients may present with lesions on the extremities such as hands and feet or even on the thighs and arms in the elderly. This is more common than tongue or mouth ulcers (Williams *et al.*, 1984).

In summary, it can be said that pemphigus is a dangerous progressive disorder of the skin whereas, pemphigoid is more common, more a disease of the tongue and mouth, and runs a benign course.

Amyloidosis of a primary nature is a rare disorder presenting with a so-called woody tongue, and sometimes macroglossia.

Dermatitis herpetiformis appears to be a very rare sensitivity reaction of unknown aetiology but associated with circulating immune complexes and occurring in certain tissue types. Although important in gastroenterology because of association with gluten enteropathy, changes in the gut and small bowel, and oral and tongue lesions are described as occurring (Fraser *et al.*, 1973). However, our recent ten-year search of records of tongue lesions revealed no recently reported cases.

222 Small discrete vesicles on the tongue tip due to Herpes simplex infection.

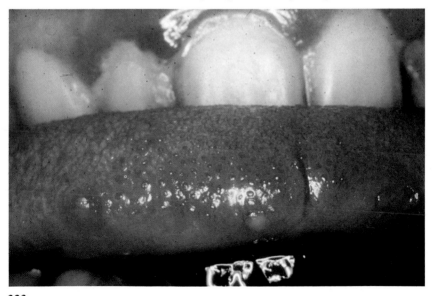

222

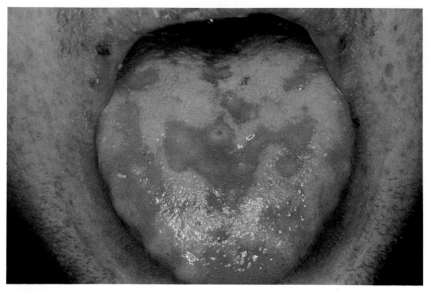

223

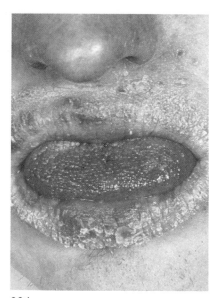

223 Erythema multiforme on the tongue secondary to sulphonamide in a young male.

224 Healing stages of Stevens-Johnson syndrome in a young Down's syndrome patient.

224

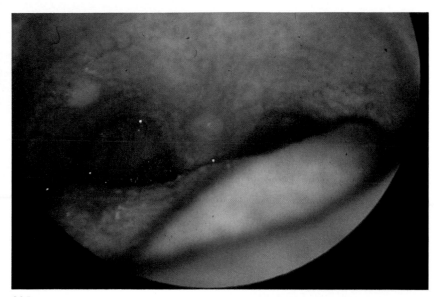

225

225 Acute Stevens-Johnson syndrome with small bullae on soft palate and coated white tongue.

226 Infectious mononucleosis with secondary drug reaction to amoxycillin. These reactions are also seen with cytomegaloviral infections and amoxycillin.

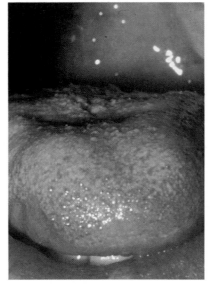

226

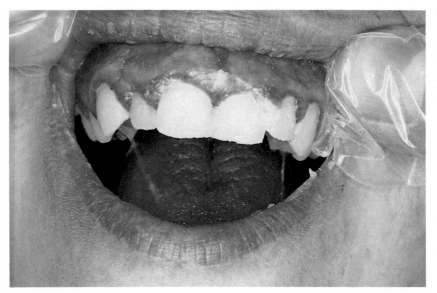

227

227 Acute drug eruption with bullous lesion on the gingiva and acute glossitis. No obvious bullae on the tongue.

228 Pemphigoid lesions along the edge of the tongue.

229 Pemphigoid of the tongue secondary to gastro-intestinal malignancy.

230 Marked pemphigoid posterior tongue.

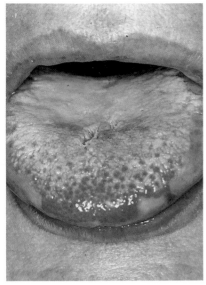

228

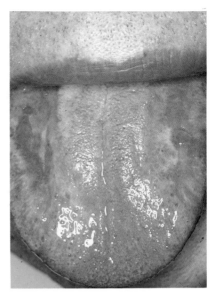

229

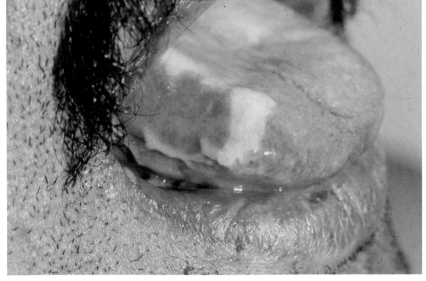

230

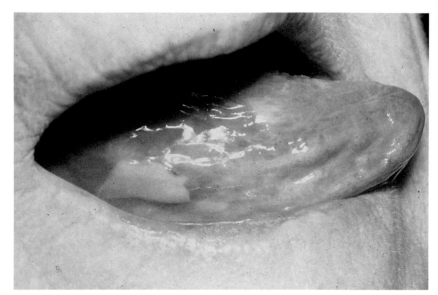

231

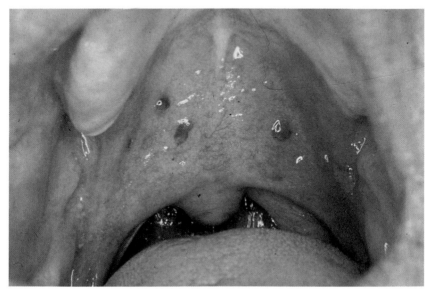

232

146

231 Unusual pemphigoid along the tongue edge in an elderly woman.

232 Pemphigus vulgaris mainly on the hard palate but some spots posteriorly on the left tongue.

233 Pemphigus of the tongue. This is always a very serious disease and can be life-threatening.

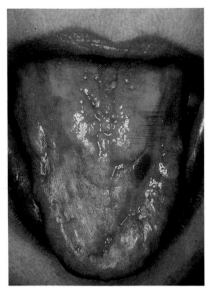

233

References

Anderson W.A.D., Kissane J.M. (Eds). Pathology of the tongue. In: *Pathology*. C.V. Mosby, St Louis, 1984, Vol 2, Ch 29.

Fraser N.G., Kerr N.W., Donald D. Oral lesions in dermatitis herpetiformis. *Br J Dermatology* 1973, **89**, 439-450.

Lynch D.P. Ulcerations of the tongue. Clinical manifestations of mucocutaneous and vesiculo-ulcerative diseases. *Postgrad Med* 1984, **75**(4), 191-203.

Williams D.M., Leonard J.M., Wright P. *et al*. Benign mucous membrane (cicatricial) pemphigoid revisited: A clinical and immunological reappraisal. *Br Dental J* 1984, **157**, 313-316.

Chapter 13
Specific Disease and Surface Lesions

Whitish appearances on the tongue reflect hyperkeratosis and the diffusion of light by keratohyalin granules (Tyldesley, 1974). Some authors also report increased hydration of this thickened keratin layer. This can almost be likened to the whiteness which appears in the skin of the feet when they are left too long lying in the bath! Whiteness can also be caused by diffuse coating in association with anaemia, and in diffuse candida of the tongue. Where vesicles and bullae of the tongue are present they may collapse down to give a whitish appearance. In lesions of lichen planus, white areas may appear, especially if there is any accompanying chronic ulceration. Krull *et al.* (1973) maintain that 5-10% of oral malignancies present as white keratotic lesions.

Any suspicion requires a suitable biopsy, but above all, early detection and referral to specialists, saving tongue function and perhaps life. Sometimes a distinction is drawn between keratotic and non-keratotic lesions of the mouth – the latter almost always of short duration and being associated with erosion, ulceration or bullae.

Frictional keratoses. Transient habit inclusion of inner cheek between the occlusive surfaces of the teeth. Sometimes seen on the lips but not the tongue.

Tobacco keratoses. Previously seen more in association with pipe-smoking with the palate usually affected, but the tongue is rarely involved. The lesions may be nicotine-stained.

Leukoplakia of the tongue. 'Leukoplakia is currently used as a clinical descriptive term for a range of non-specific white lesions of the oral mucosa – from slightly raised, white, translucent areas to dense, white, opaque lesions with or without adjacent ulceration, to speckled site with interspersed areas of erosion or ulceration' (Shklar, 1986).

Small white areas which could be defined as leukoplakia, but where the lesion is small and a biopsy negative may slowly fade. Small lesions on the dorsum of the tongue, as mentioned above, have a low rate of malignancy but up to 20% of persistent lesions on the under-surface of the tongue in older age groups may show malignant changes.

This complex topic is well reviewed from Harvard in an editiorial in which the relative rarity of lesions on the tongue is noted (only 8.5%) when compared with the commisurae or buccal mucosa (26%). However, ventral lingual lesions appear to be particularly prone to malignant transformation (Kramer, 1980). Although more commonly described in men than women by about three to one, some observers suggest an increasing incidence in women. As the only effective current treatment should be in the hands of an oral medicine specialist, early referral for opinion, observation or biopsy of lesions is important.

The World Health Organization's definition of leukoplakia is a clinical description: '*A white patch which cannot be rubbed off and is not due to any identifiable cause*'. These lesions are produced by a variety of disorders (Kramer, 1980).

An experienced observer (i.e. an oral medicine consultant) will recognise a high percentage of lesions and interpret the cytology. Amongst the more commonly seen areas of leukoplakia are: dyskeratotic lesions; squamous carcinoma *in situ* (edges of lichen planus?). As Kramer has summed it up, 'We must avoid thinking about leukoplakia as a particular disease until we have more understanding of its origins and nature'.

Lichen planus. McCarthy and Shklar (1980) review well the tongue lesions of this disorder of characteristic appearances but unknown aetiology. They describe a group of patterns which others do not always recognise.

A *Striated pattern* 'lace-like' (so-called striae).

B *Atrophic pattern.* With time the white lesions give way to a thinning of the epithelium and a true atrophic glossitis. Eventually the lichen planus slowly disappears to give the reddened tongue of chronic glossitis.

C *Erosive or ulcerative.* These can be small erosions and a general reticular pattern, or rarely larger ulcers with or without secondary bacterial infection. The 'malignant' types are seen in the wider erosive forms.

D *Plaque pattern.* This is described as affecting the central dorsum and lips rather than the common lichen planus sites of the edges of the tongue. Affected areas seem more grey and sunken due to atrophy below, leaving surrounding filiforms more intact. Histopathology, ultrasound and differential diagnosis are specialised topics and well reviewed by McCarthy and Shklar (1980).

Other specific lesions of the tongue's dorsal surface (Arndt, 1971) include the following.

Patches of radiation injury (where the clinical history is important).

Hereditary avascular lesions

Psoriasis (tongue is never affected without at least small patches on elbows, knees, fingernails or scalp) (Dawson, 1974).

Syphilis (now unusual and confirmed on biopsy and on serology).

Chronic discoid lupus (uncommon in the absence of other skin lesions, especially on palms or soles).

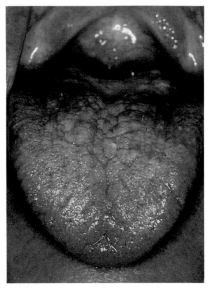

234

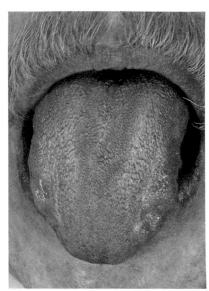

235

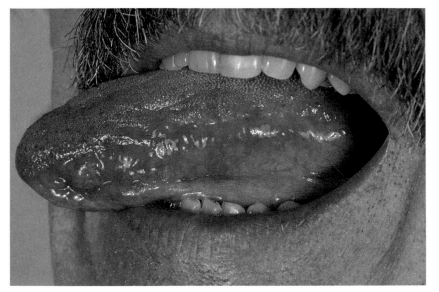

236

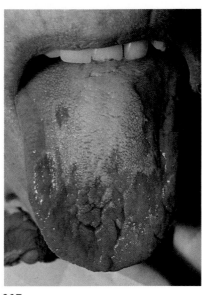

234 Tobacco keratoses in a 61-year-old driver. Differential diagnosis lichen planus or leukoplakia.

235 Early leukoplakia in a 42-year-old non-smoking male doctor. Only the left edge of the tongue is involved.

236 An area of leukoplakia on the mid-left edge has been surgically removed but very small areas of early leukoplakia are still present.

237 An area of leukoplakia and super-infection with candidiasis in an 80-year-old housewife.

237

Systemic sclerosis (the tongue may be relatively immobile and shrunken without much involvement on the surface).

Sarcoidosis (rare for tongue surface to be involved without mediastinal involvement).

Chronic patchy glossitis (this can occur with a relatively patchy appearance in some patients on chronic medication.

Pityriasis (often diagnosed as chronic glossitis).

Main causes
A Acute or chronic drug glossitis
B Lichen planus
C Leukoplakia
D Radiation injury

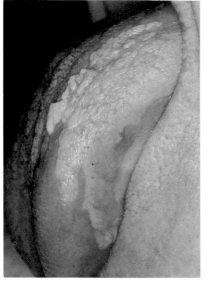

238

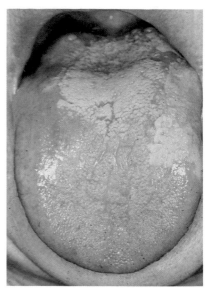

239

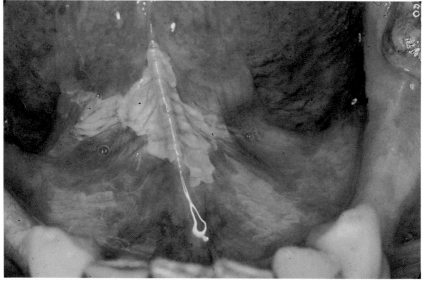

240

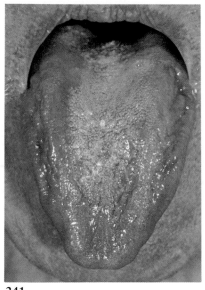
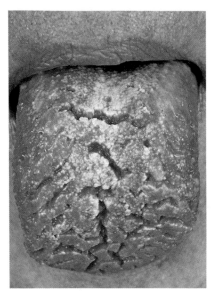

241
242

238 An area of leukoplakia on the dorsum of the tongue of a middle-aged negroid seaman.

239 Patchy leukoplakia of an elderly woman.

240 A discrete patch of leukoplakia underneath the tongue.

241 Mild central leukoplakia shading into a heavy coating on the tongue of an elderly woman.

242 Candida infection masquerading as leukoplakia in a deeply fissured tongue.

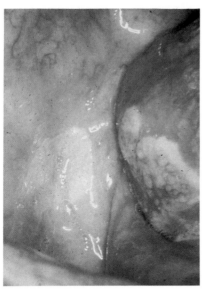

243   Small isolated patches of leukoplakia on the side of the tongue and buccal mucosa.

244   Indurated and eroded area of leukoplakia with a possible diagnosis of erosive lichen planus or carcinoma *in situ*. A biopsy showed only dyskeratotic lesions.

245 and 246   Localised patches of leukoplakia on the right side of the tongue in an elderly man. Biopsy of the area under the tongue and on the lateral border revealed carcinoma.

243

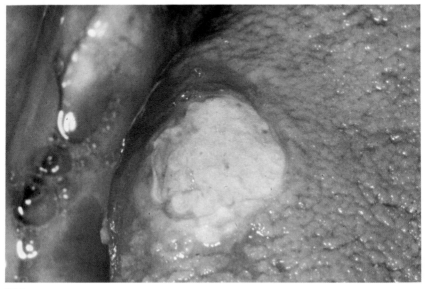

244

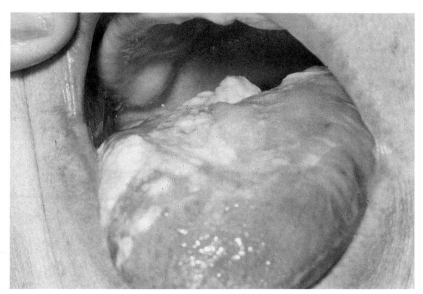

245

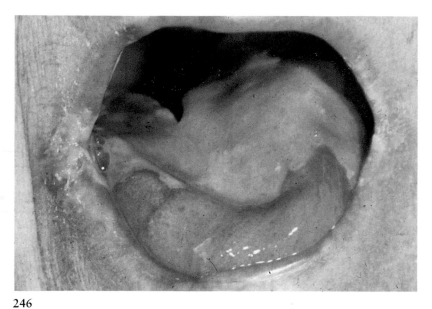

246

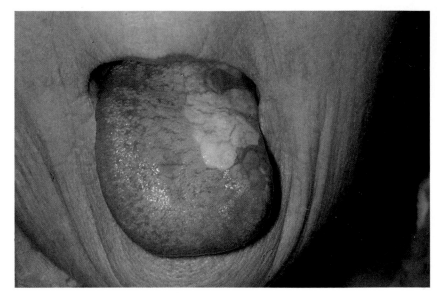

247

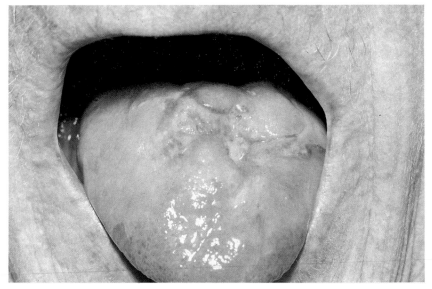

248

156

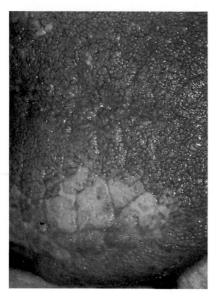

249

247 Isolated plaques of leukoplakia in an elderly woman with no other known disorder. No carcinoma *in situ* on biopsy.

248 Extensive areas of leukoplakia thought to be due to trauma. Biopsy of the left edge of the tongue showed carcinoma *in situ*.

249 Acute glossitis with a white patch thought to be leukoplakia but eventually diagnosed as lichen planus.

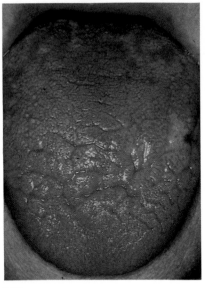 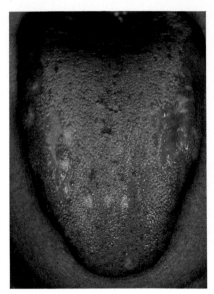

250   251

250   Small area of lichen planus on the right side of the tongue.

251   More extensive lichen planus with diffuse coating of the tongue and emphasis on fungiforms.

252   Lichen planus on the edge of the tongue.

253   More marked lichen planus showing a lateral border of the tongue.

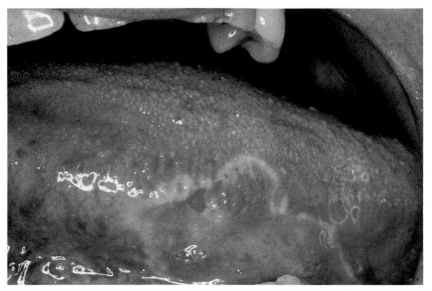

252

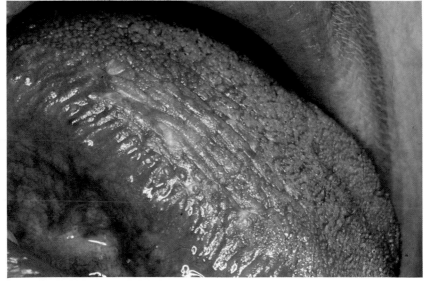

253

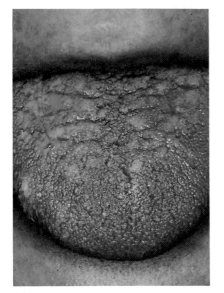

254

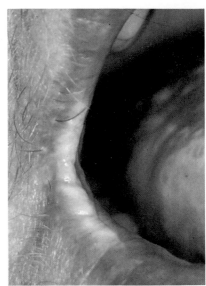

255

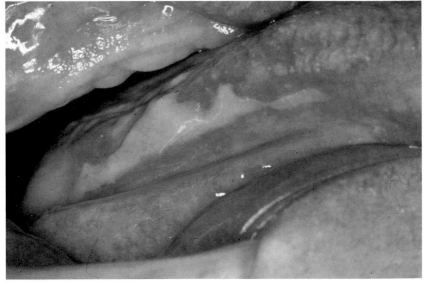

256

254 More extensive lichen planus covering the whole dorsum and spreading onto the ventral surface of the tongue.

255 Lichen planus showing involvement of the lip edge (a frequent clinical marker) as well as on the tongue.

256 Lichen planus predominantly along the edge of the tongue beginning to show erosive features.

257 Lichen planus with patchy semi-plaque-like patterns.

258 Lichen planus under the left side of the tongue.

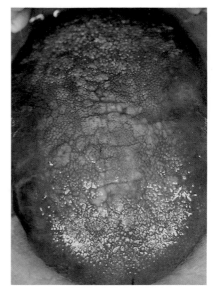

257

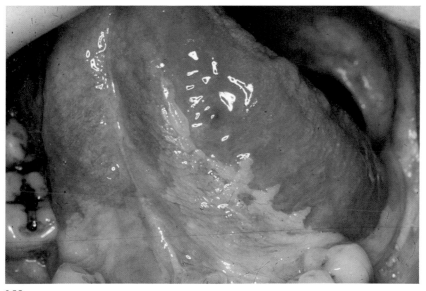

258

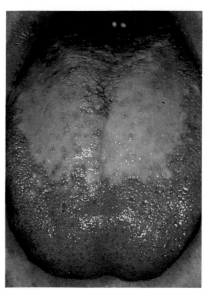

259 Atrophic features of lichen planus developing near the tip of the tongue with thinning of the epithelium.

260 Lichen planus on gums of negroid patient (desquamative gingivitis).

259

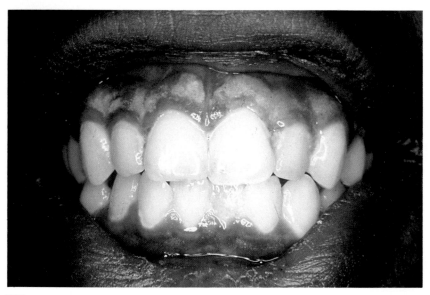

260

261 Widespread lichen planus with some striated patterns on the dorsum of the tongue.

262 A pattern of lichen planus on the ventral surface of the tongue but sparing the frenum.

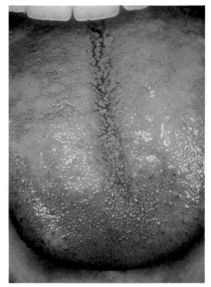

261

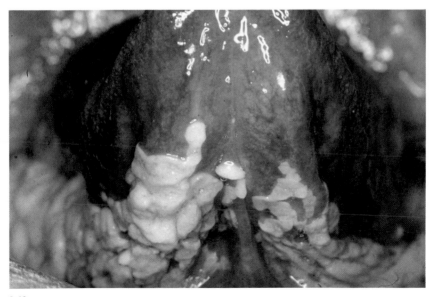

262

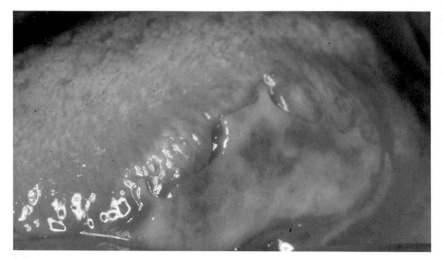

263

263 Erosive form of lichen planus, along lateral border of the tongue. Bacterial over-growth needs to be excluded.

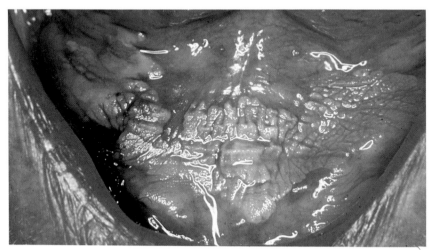

264

264 Lichen planus under the tongue with small patches of erosion especially on the right.

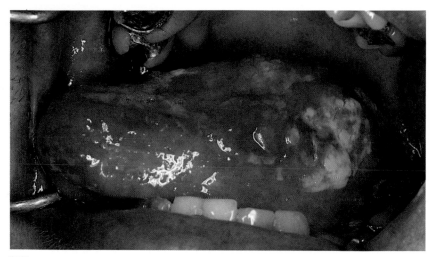

265

265 Erosive lichen planus on the left lateral edge of the tongue with ulcerative features. Biopsy of persistent ulceration showed cancerous changes.

References

Arndt K. Lichen planus. In *Dermatology in General Medicine*. Fitzgerald T.B. (Ed.) McGraw-Hill, New York, 1971, pp728-735.

Banoczy J. *Oral Leukoplakia*. Martinus Nijhoff, The Hague, 1982.

Dawson T.A.J. Tongue lesions in generalised pustular psoriasis. *Br J Dermatol* 1974, **91**, 419-424.

Kramer I.R.H. Editorial. Oral leukoplakia. *J Roy Soc Med* 1980, **73**, 765-67.

Krull E.A., Fellman A.C., Fabian L.A. White lesions of the mouth. *Clinical Symposia* 1973, **25**, 2-32.

McCarthy P.L., Shklar G. *Dieseases of Oral Mucosa*, 2nd edn. Lea & Febiger, Philadelphia, 1980 pp203-224.

Scully C., El-Kom M. Lichen planus: review and update on pathogenesis. *J Oral Path* 1985, **14**, 431-458.

Shklar G. Oral Leukoplakia. An Editorial review. *New Engl J Med* 1986, **315**, 1544-1545.

Tyldesley W.R. Oral lesions in diseases of the skin. *Br Dental J* 1974, **136**, 23-27.

Waldron C.A. Shafer W.G. Leukoplakia revisited: A clinicopathologic study of 3256 oral leukoplakias. *Cancer* 1975, **36**, 1386-1392.

Chapter 14

Infections

Most infections of the tongue are also seen in the oral mucous membrane, the gingiva and sometimes the skin. At an early stage, various fungal infections may be confined to the crypts between the filiform papillae, and candidiasis can also be confined to a single area of the tongue. The most common tongue infections are candidiasis or 'thrush' in the elderly, in those who have received steroids or antibiotics, in poorly controlled diabetics or in those with reduced resistance to infection. Thus, patients undergoing therapy for leukaemia or other neoplastic conditions and those having suppression of graft reactions or autoimmune disorders are particularly susceptible (Main *et al.*, 1984; Samaranayake *et al.*, 1984).

The presence of viral bacterial or fungal infections must always raise questions about humoral and tissue resistance. If no obvious general pathology is present the whole question of nutritional and alcohol status should be explored and an Elisa and western blot test for HIV antibodies using serum should be done. Histoplasma granuloma occurs with septicaemic infection and disseminated histoplasmosis.

The most common childhood xanthema of measles and chickenpox can give rise to lesions on the tongue although this is more often spared, even when Koplik spots may be seen in the buccal mucosa.

14.1 Viral infections

Herpes simplex: more often on the lip margin (Grattan *et al.*, 1986; Milacic, 1980).

Herpes varicella zoster: almost always skin lesions on mandibular division of the face.

Herpes simplex: also seen in other immune compromised states (Ogilvie *et al.*, 1983).

Epstein-Barr: infectious mononucleosis (there is also the rare association with Burkitt lymphoma).

Coxsackie B infections.

14.2 Bacterial infections

These seldom affect the tongue alone and are now rarely seen in 'western-style' living. Here, immunisation for diphtheria and whooping cough and the widespread use of penicillin derivatives have greatly reduced indigenous streptococcal populations with a reduction in scarlet fever and the 'strawberry' tongue.

Rare conditions of the mouth, seldom seen in the tongue are:

Tuberculosis (Dimtrowa *et al.*, 1981).

Actinomycosis.

Histoplasmosis (due to *H. capsulatum*).

Cysticerosis (Lustmann & Copelyn, 1981).

Donovanosis (due to *Calymmatobacterum granulomatosis*).

Secondary bacterial infections with staphylococci, *Streptococcus faecalis* and coliform and gram-negative bacilli can be cultured from tongue ulcers in debilitated patients, in radio-necrotic areas of the tongue and after reconstructive surgery to the tongue.

14.3 Fungal infections

Candidiasis of the tongue is common (Shepherd, 1982; Shepherd *et al.*, 1983, 1985) and gives white patches due to growth of the yeast *Candida albicans*. One classification of oral thrush is as follows.

A Acute   Pseudomembranous thrush
Atrophic candidiasis (secondary to antibiotic stomatitis)

B Chronic   Atrophic secondary to denture wearing
Hyperplastic as in chronic hyperplastic candidiasis

C Chronic   mucocutaneous candidiasis

Less commonly, fusospirochaetal infections from gingival ulceration may spread onto the root or posterior of the tongue. This is produced by a spirochaete, *Treponema vincentii* acting with *Fusobacterium* species, particularly *necrophorum*.

Other more unusual mycoses can affect the tongue in debilitated or immunosuppressed patients (Trotoux *et al.*, 1982).

14.4 Sexually transmitted infections

As syphilitic ulcers and plaques of the tongue are seen less and less (Malik *et al.*, 1983), the small ulcers secondary to Reiter's syndrome are becoming increasingly common. Herpetic ulcerations, acute candidiasis and Kaposi's sarcoma lesions can all be a presenting feature on the tongue of the retrovirus HIV (Marcusen & Sooy, 1985). In most tongue infections, other lesions can be found during a careful examination of the oral mucous membrane or gingiva.

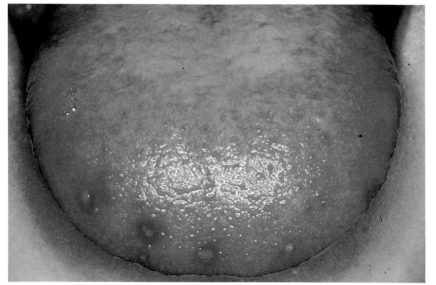

266

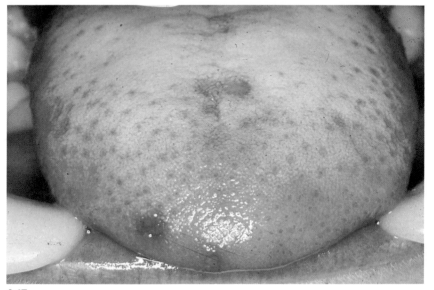

267

266 Herpetic stomatitis confined to the tongue of a 21-year-old female clerk.

267 Febrile coating of the tongue with two herpetic lesions at the tip.

268 Herpetic lesions with secondary infection and acute glossitis on the dorsum of the tongue in a middle-aged woman.

269 Geographic tongue appearance developing in a young nurse with Epstein-Barr infection (mononucleosis). Febrile illness and sore throat associated with ulceration of tonsillar tissue and petechial haemorrhages.

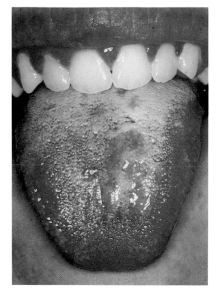

268

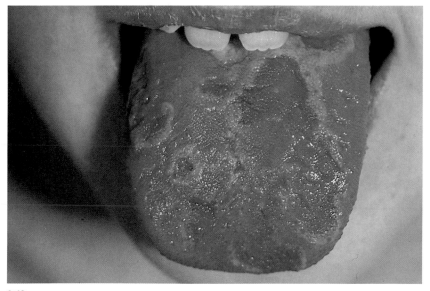

269

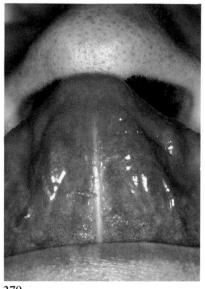
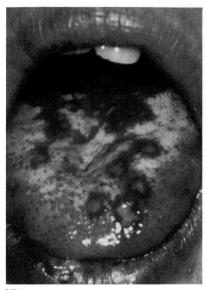

270

271

270　Herpetic lesions around the tip and on the left side of the tongue of a child with the appearance of small warty lesions.

271　Herpes simplex infection (Type 2) – lips and tongue.

272　Very unusual appearances of Burkitt's lymphoma. This 43-year-old woman had travelled widely but not in Africa. Epstein-Barr virus and cytology confirmed the diagnosis.

273　Herpes zoster infection or shingles (chickenpox virus) with right facial palsy. The unilateral lesion is commonly described in H2 infections but the demarcation shown is very marked.

274　Herpes zoster or shingles with the Ramsay-Hunt syndrome involvement of facial nerve and auditory nerve branch with vesicles in external ear and some hearing loss and facial palsy.

275　Diffuse candidiasis in an elderly man with newly diagnosed diabetes mellitus.

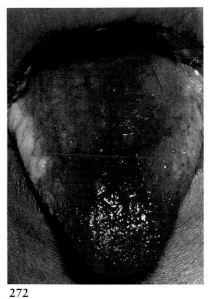

272

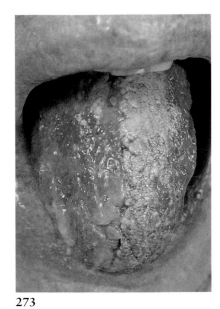

273

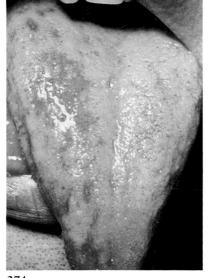

274

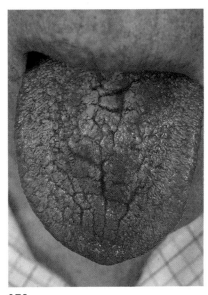

275

276 Strawberry tongue with haemolytic streptococcus and 'scarlet fever'.

277 Unusual tongue appearances from 69-year-old man with a long history of diabetes mellitus. Poor nutrition from alcohol excess, some smoking and chronic left ventricular failure. Note cyanotic hue. Admitted with acute diabetic hyperglycaemia and *Candida albicans* grown from dorsum of the tongue and palate.

278 Small patches of candidiasis in a young girl with generalised autoimmune disorder, probably systemic lupus erythematosis.

279 Diffuse candidiasis infection in 80-year-old nutritionally deficient, edentulous widow living alone. Positive fungal swabs followed a short course of tetracycline.

280 Widespread thrush in 50-year-old wasted Polynesian male with combined tuberculosis and diabetes.

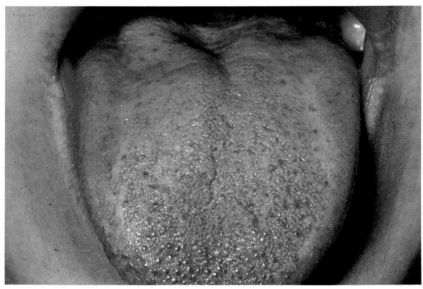

276

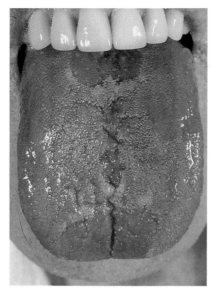

277

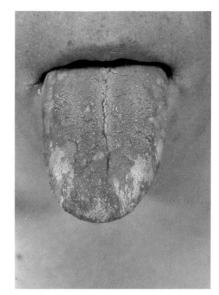

278

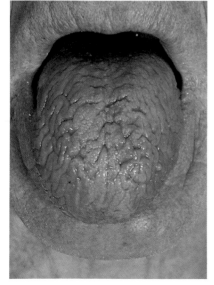

279

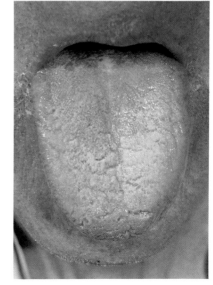

280

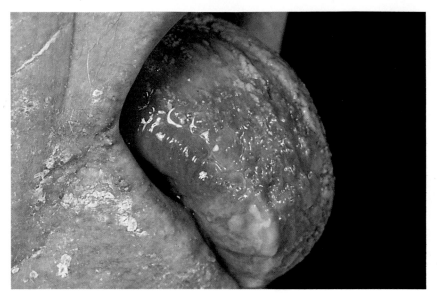

281

281 Lateral view of the tongue of elderly woman with Herpes zoster and superimposed candidiasis of the tongue.

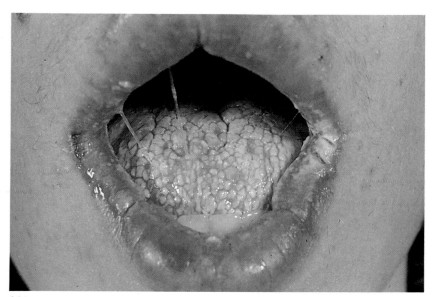

282

282 Young boy with severe endocrine autoimmune disorder. Acute pseudomembranous thrush after a course of tetracyclines.

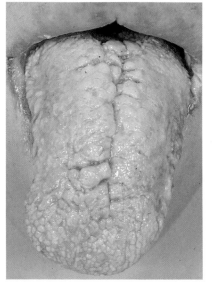

283

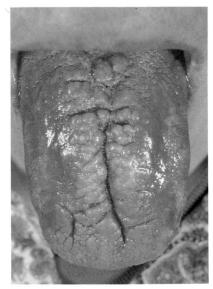

284

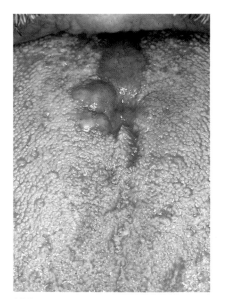

285

283 and 284 Brother of former patient (**282**), also with multiple autoimmune disease on corticosteroids for Addison's disease replacement, shows widespread pseudomembranous candidiasis.
Two weeks after successful treatment by local and general amphotericin therapy.

285 Widespread *Candida* infection on a hairy tongue with some normal mid-line variation.

286 and 287 A 74-year-old retired carpenter with diabetes mellitus, undergoing surgery for cancer of the bowel, developed severe pseudomembranous thrush after being given steroids. Mixed bacterial and fungal infection with patches also seen on the soft palate.

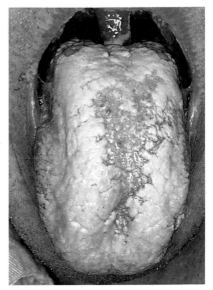

286

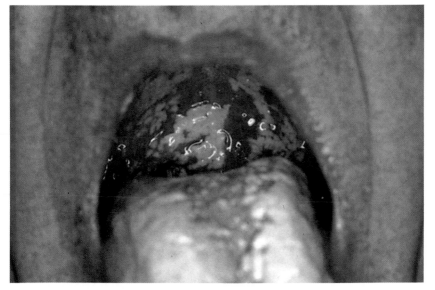

287

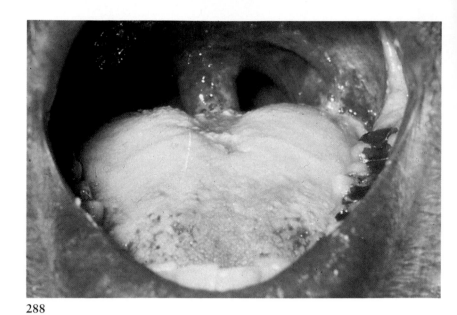

288

288 Extreme example of pseudomembranous candidiasis.

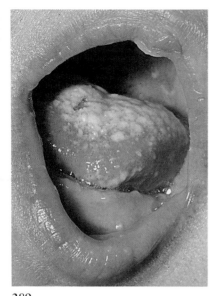

289

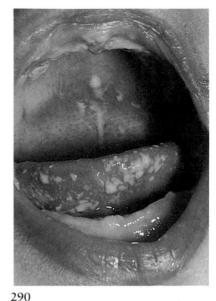

290

289 and 290 Infant with pseudo-membranous disease on the tongue and palate with widespread buccal and gingival involvement, and also fusiform infection. Immune suppression disorder.

291 Teenage girl with acute glossitis with patches of thrush due to *Candida*.

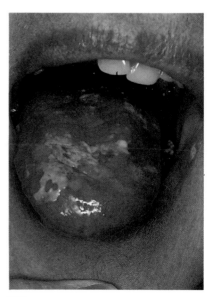

291

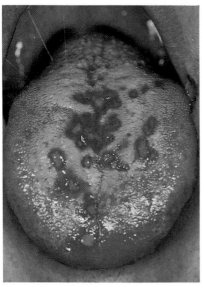

292 20-year-old sailor presenting with widespread Herpes simplex infections of the tongue, now showing widespread secondary candidiasis. HIV antibody negative but immune status reduced for unknown reasons.

293 18-year-old male student with symptoms of Reiter's disease and 'sore' mouth with a small erosive lesion on the lateral border of the tongue and vesicles on the anterior pillar of the fauces.

292

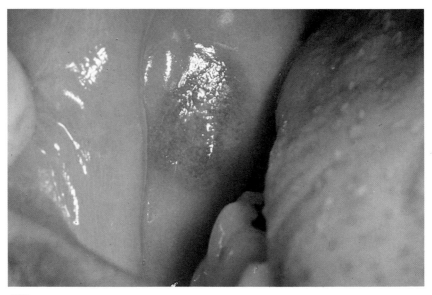

293

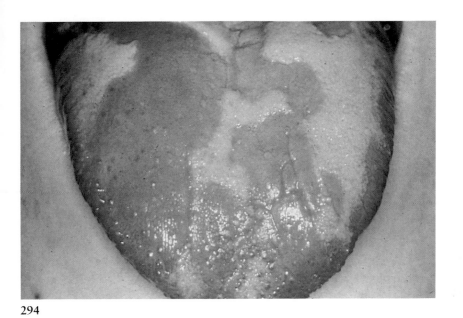

294

294 Unusual Reiter's disease of tongue and secondary candidiasis.

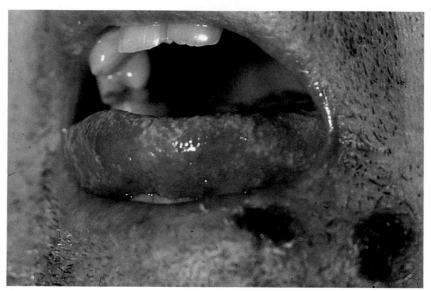

295

295 Herpetic ulceration and *Candida* infection in a man who is immuno-suppressed for renal transplant.

296 and 297 Patchy *Candida* infection along both lateral borders of the tongue in a 28-year-old night-club attendant. Swabs positive for *Candida* and serum positive for HIV virus and HTLV III antibody.

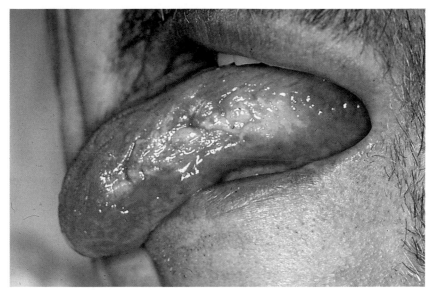

296

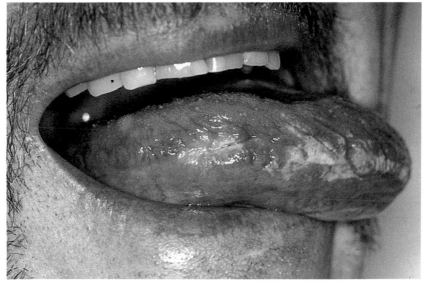

297

183

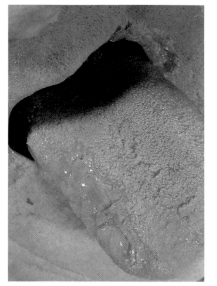

298

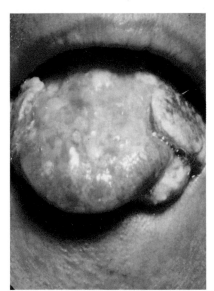

299

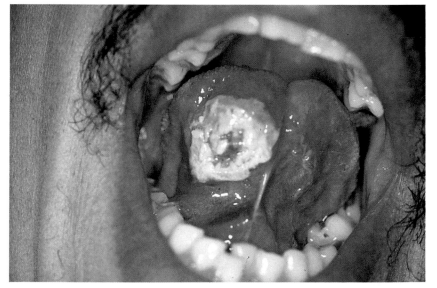

300

298 60-year-old male international marine engineer with coating of the tongue and epithelial plaques along the right border. Serology and biopsy confirm diagnosis of secondary syphilis.

299 Tongue showing interstitial glossitis of syphilitic gumma (tertiary syphilis) together with a squamous cell carcinoma.

300 The very rare condition of syphilitic chancroid under the tongue.

References

Dimitrowa I., Bajdekow B., Balabanowa M. Tuberculosis of the tongue (author's translation). *Z Hautkr* 1981, 56(4), 221-226.

Grattan C.E.H., Small D., Kennedy C.T.C. *et al*. Oral herpes simplex infection in bullous pemphigoid. *Oral Surg Oral Med Oral Pathol* 1986, **61**, 40-43.

Lustmann J., Copelyn M. Oral cysticercosis. A review of the literature and report of two cases. *Int J Oral Surg* 1981, 10(5), 371-375.

Main B.E., Calman K.C., Ferguson M.M. Kaye S.B., *et al*. The effect of cytotoxic therapy on saliva and oral flora. *Oral Surg* 1984, **58**, 545.

Malik P.A., Cabbabe E.B., Shively R.E. *et al*. Condyloma acuminatum of the tongue. *Ann Plastic Surg* 1983, **10**, 417-420.

Marcusen D.C., Sooy C.D. Otolaryngologic and head and neck manifestations of acquired immuno-deficiency syndrome (AIDS). *Laryngoscope* 1985, **95**, 401-405.

Ogilvie M.M., Kessler M., Leppard B.J. *et al*. Herpes simplex infections in pemphigus: An indication for urgent viral studies and specific antiviral therapy. *Br J Dermat* 1983, **109**, 611-613.

Samaranayake L.P., Calman K.C., Ferguson M.M. *et al*. The oral carriage of yeast and coliforms in patients on cytotoxic therapy. *J Oral Path* 1984, **13**, 390.

Shepherd M.G. 'Candidiasis' – An infectious disease of increasing importance. *NZ Dent J* 1982, **78**, 89-93.

Shepherd M.G., Smith J.M.B., Sullivan P.A. *et al*. 'Candidiasis'. *NZ Med J* 1983, **96**, 612-619.

Shepherd M.G., Poulter R.T.M., Sullivan P.A. *Candida albicans*: Biology, genetics and pathogenicity. *Ann Review Microbiol* 1985, **39**, 579-614.

Trotoux J., Dupont B., Drouhet E. Mycotic lingual granuloma. The pseudotumoral form. *Ann Otolaryngol Chir Cervicofac* 1982, **99**(12), 553-556.

Chapter 15

Colour Changes

A mild coating will often produce a white tongue, widely seen in all patients feeling too unwell to eat. Other colours of the tongue may have quite common associations. A good example would be a blue tongue seen in disorders giving rise to central cyanosis. Many heart and lung diseases might, in their later stages, lead to blood perfusing unoxygenated areas of the lung because of fluid, fibrosis or shunting. As long as 5 g/dl of haemoglobin can be reduced, a faint bluish cyanosis will be seen on the tongue.

The blueness of the tongue can thus be valuable because many conditions may produce slowed blood flow at the extremities and therefore have reduced haemoglobin, but a blue tongue, seen against a normal-coloured skin, indicated central cyanosis. Other coloured tongues likewise have specific associations. A list of colours and the likely clinical signs or history and possible diagnoses are set out in Table 9 which provides a quick check on possible causes for the colour changes.

Whilst it is clearly not possible to make diagnoses from an observation of the colour of the tongue, such observations are a training in clinical methodology. The recognition by such training of pattern or colour is emphasised to alert the primary health worker or non-specialist in mouth disease to a need for more careful examination. Thus, colour can be an important indicator for health workers.

Table 9 Conditions associated with abnormally coloured tongues

Colour	Common association	Look also for
Pale yellow	Anaemia Jaundice	Glossitis Fetor Spider naevi Dupuytren's contracture of palms Liver palms (erythema)
Orange	Obstructive jaundice	A combination of coated tongue, mild jaundice and nutritional deficiencies
Strawberry red	Scarlet fever Antibiotics 'Pernicious' anaemia (B12 deficiency) Sprue	Tonsillitis Diarrhoea Palpable liver and spleen Neurology Abdominal tenderness
Blue	Cyanosis Polycythaemia Raynaud's disease	Lung disease Congenital heart disease Palpable spleen High platelets Blue/white changes, also severe in extremities (Guinta, 1975)
Beefy red	B vitamin deficiency	Cheilosis
Magenta	Aribinoflavinosis	Nutritional deficiencies (especially in the gingiva)
Pigmented	Can be racial Addison's disease Heroin addiction Malignant melanoma Thyroid	Hypotension Low serum Na and high K Needle sites in arms (Westerhof et al., 1983) (Jlanner et al., 1980) Palpable or enlarged gland Tremor of fingers Eye signs
Black (hairy)	Metal poisoning	Smoking, poor oral hygiene Industrial or 'hobby' history

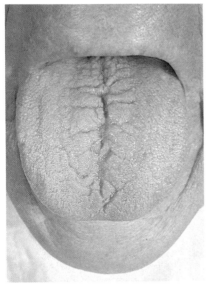

301

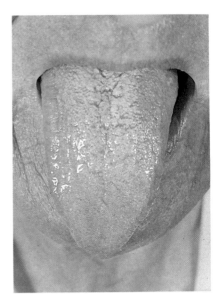

302

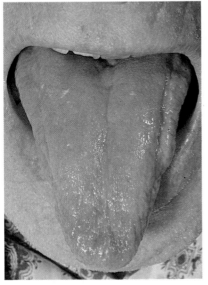

303

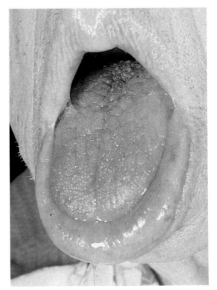

304

188

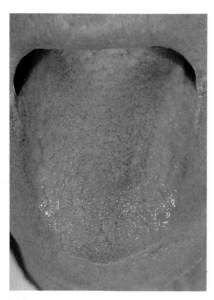

305

301 82-year-old woman with marked folate deficient anaemia and largish white tongue suggesting hypothyroidism with coexistant anaemia. Thyroid indices were reduced.

302 Pale tongue from nutritional anaemia in a 79-year-old ex-soldier living alone. Whiteness exaggerated by diffuse superficial *Candida* infection or candidiasis.

303 81-year-old man with mild Vitamin B12 deficiency, untreated pernicious anaemia and pale pink-white tongue.

304 Pale pink tongue of an 83-year-old woman. Blood and bone marrow examinations confirm gross Vitamin B12 deficiency. Note atrophy of the edge of the tongue consistent with gastric atrophy. Her three sisters have pernicious anaemia.

305 Pale fawn tongue of a middle-aged man of mixed racial origin. Colour due to a combination of mild cyanosis due to chronic lung disease, anaemia and smoking.

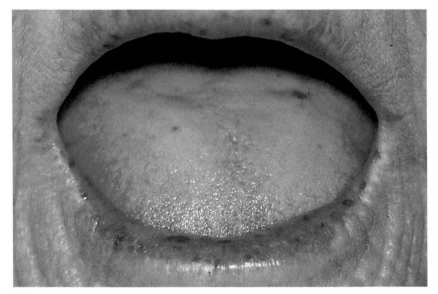

306

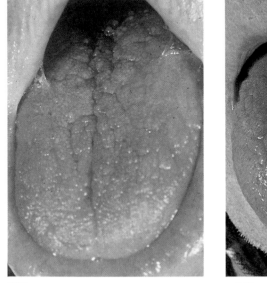

307

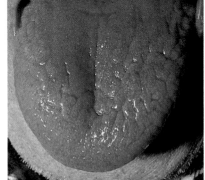

308

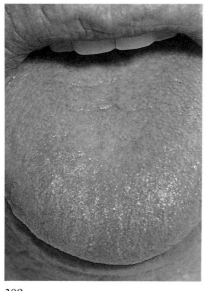 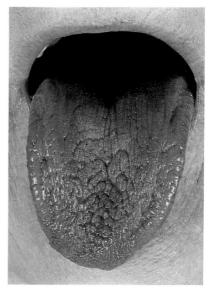

309   310

306   Very mild jaundice secondary to systemic sclerosis.

307   Pale orange-yellow tongue due to combined anaemia and very mild jaundice in a 69-year-old woman undergoing biliary duct surgery.

308   Orange tongue in 68-year-old retired postal worker. Colour due to combined anaemia and *Candida*.

309   70-year-old housewife with lilac-pink tongue secondary to mild glossitis, possibly of chemical origin.

310   Bright red tongue of a 61-year-old countrywoman with chronic diarrhoea secondary to prolonged course of antibiotics. Acute atrophic candidiasis of the tongue.

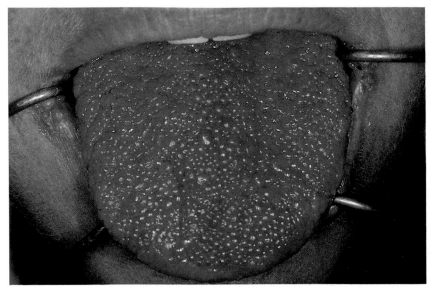

311

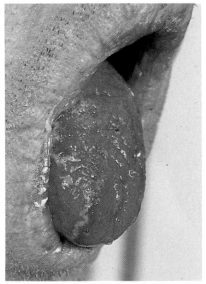

312

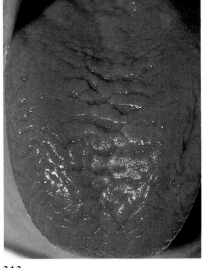

313

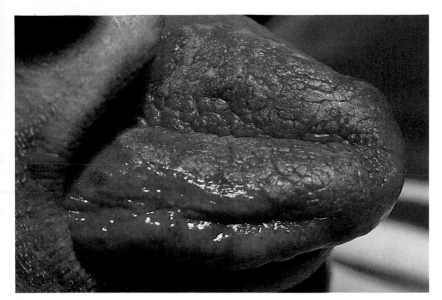

314

311 Very acute painful glossitis with a bright, berry-like red tongue related to nutritional deficiencies (i.e. documented B vitamin).

312 Prematurely aged unemployed alcoholic male of 55 years with acute glossitis secondary to multiple Vitamin B deficiencies.

313 A beefy red tongue secondary to acute B vitamin deficiency.

314 Lateral view of beefy red tongue showing some glossitis in an alcoholic negro.

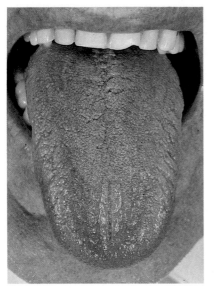

315

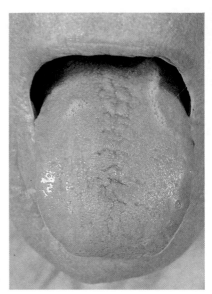

316

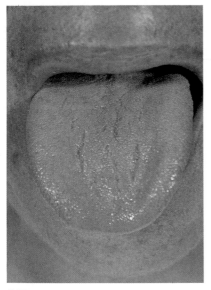

317

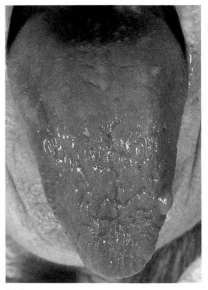

318

194

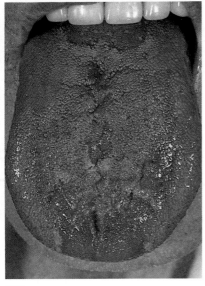
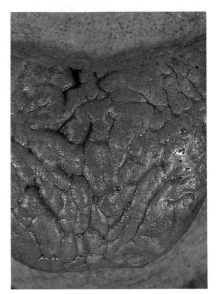

319   320

315   Red tongue of glossitis with a hint of cyanosis (PAO$_2$ reduced) in retired clerk given antibiotics for bronchitis.

316   Magenta tongue with very mild filiform atrophy and mild cyanosis, Riboflavin deficiency identified from dietary survey.

317   Pale mauve tongue in middle-aged Indian woman with chronic bronchitis, antibiotic treatment (penicillin and tetracyclines), mild glossitis and mild cyanosis.

318   Dark mauve tongue seen in edentulous old lady with increase in size of the tongue because of a lax frenum and lack of dentures. Note also the mild glossitis, probably from her oxyphenbutazone and carbamezine.

319   Large pale purple tongue in hypothyroid patient admitted to hospital with chronic lung disease and slight left stroke.

320   Unusual purple tongue with extensive fissures, mild glossitis and blue coating. Polypharmacy with seven medications which included thiazide diuretics, indomethacin and naproxen.

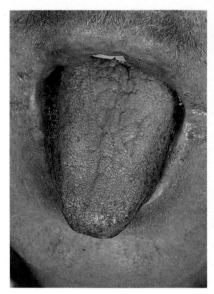

321

321 30-year-old man with dark blue tongue due to Eisenmenger complex and cardiac 'shunting'.

322 31-year-old schizophrenic patient on five high-dosage psychotropic drugs. Tongue was mildy pigmented as well as cheeks and skin, but not easily seen because of difficulties in co-operation.

323 Grey appearance of tongue produced by combination of white coating, mild cyanosis, mild anaemia and thyrotoxicosis.

324 Very brown pigmentation secondary to heavy smoking. Note also small patch of leukoplakia posteriorly. Excessive filiform hypertrophy due to poor nutrition and smoking.

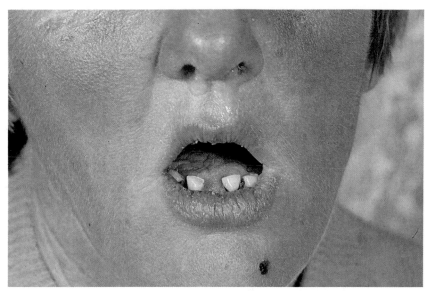

322

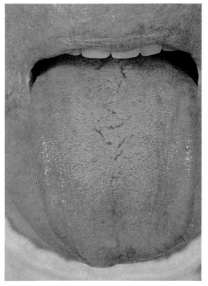

323

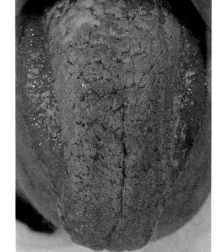

324

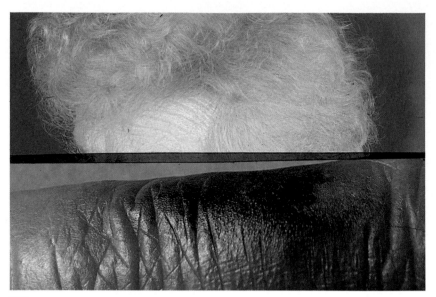

325

325 Positive smokers' sign in hair and finger.

326 Markedly positive pigmentation well seen in glossitic tongue in Russian bear-trainer.

327 Pigmented black patches in marked Addison's disease. This is relatively rarely seen today because of early treatment, the pigmented areas show up well despite the 25-year-old slide.

328 Small pigmented spots on the tongue in Addison's disease but the rare pigmentation is obvious on the buccal surface.

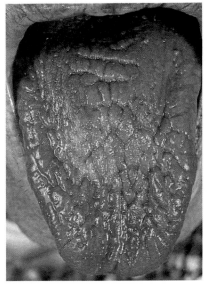

326

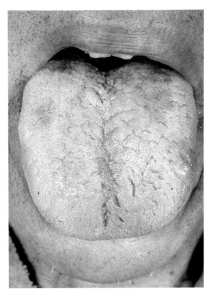

327

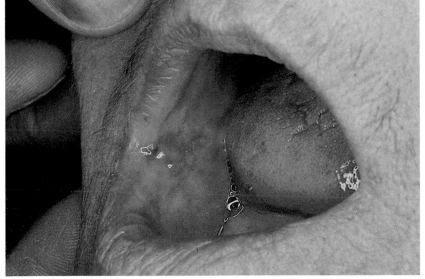

328

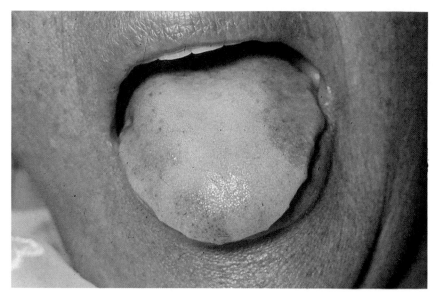

329

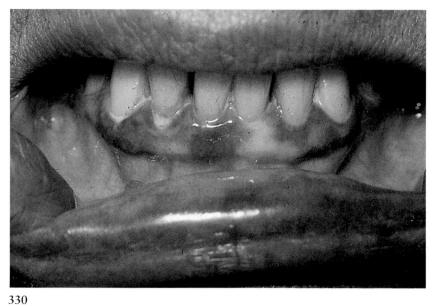

330

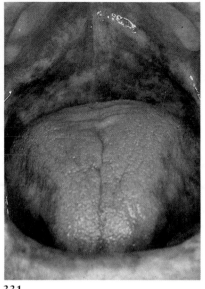

331

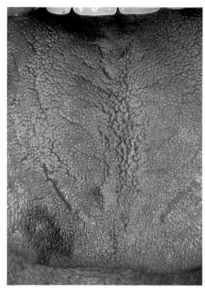

332

329 and 330 Pigmentation of racial origin in a Polynesian man with tuberculosis of lungs and adrenal glands. Also seen in gingiva.

331 Marked racial pigmentation of edges of tongue and also to some extent on roof of mouth or palate in chronically ill Maori man.

332 A single patch of pigment near the right-hand tip of the tongue in an Indian male with thyrotoxicosis.

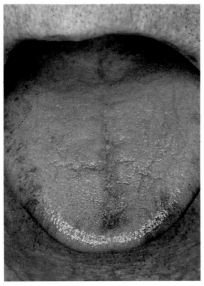 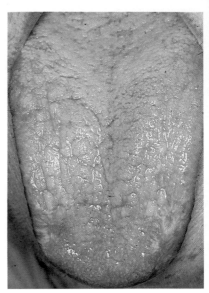

333   **334**

333   A tongue in a Polynesian man with Addison's disease.

334   Greenish-brown pigmentation in a smoker with the tongue also showing marked lichen planus.

References

Guinta J.L. Raynaud's disease with oral manifestations. *Arch Dermatol* 1975, **3**, 78-80.

Jlanner M., Marschelke I., Voigt H. Localised intramural silver impregnation of the tongue. Differential diagnosis from malignant melanoma. *Hautarzt* 1980, **31**(9), 510-512.

Westerhof W., Wolters E., Brook-Bakker J.T.W. *et al*. Pigmented lesions of the tongue in heroin addicts – fixed drug eruption. *Br J Dermatol* 1983, **109**, 605-610.

Chapter 16

Tongue Changes in Congenital and Developmental Abnormalities

16.1 Small tongue or microglossia

In the embryo, the tongue and mandible grow from the branchial arches out around the foregut opening, resulting in the development of the mouth and lips of the primitive foregut. Early arrest or delay of this regional development before the 6-8mm stage may show in the facial appearance of a small 'undershot' mandible or lower jaw, and likewise the tongue may be small. In other forms of microcephaly the mid-face may also develop slowly or imperfectly, resulting in intellectual impairment and microglossia (Boraz *et al.*, 1985). Small tongues may be seen:

as microglossia alone (slower development of speech);
as microglossia in association with microcephaly (intellectual impairment – Virchon-Siebel syndrome);
Treacher-Collins syndrome (mandibulo-facial dysostosis);
oral-facial-digital syndrome (tongue usually pitted and lobulated);
Marfan's syndrome (tongue long and thin);
Goldenhau syndrome (oculo-auricular vertebral dysplasia);
rarer disorders such as Smith-Lemli-Opitz and Coffin-Lowry syndromes (fused digits, mental retardation and osteocartilaginous disorders).

16.2 Predominantly large tongues

By far the commonest cause of the large tongues seen in association with impairment of intellect is Trisomy 21 or Down's syndrome. Here all variations of fissuring and size are seen. On occasions the tongue appears almost too big to be accommodated and is half protruded between the teeth. Absent or deficient fissuring in Down's syndrome child may suggest the possibility of cretinism or juvenile hypothyroidism. Large tongues also occur in association with a large chromosome-16. Larger than normal tongues are also seen in such rare disorders as:

Cornelia de Lange syndrome;
San Fillipo Type 3B syndrome;

Hurler's syndrome and ⎫ mucopoly saccharidosis with
Hunter's syndrome ⎭ or without gargolyism;
exophalocoele-macroglossia-gigantism syndrome (EMG or Beckwith syndrome) (Grunt & Enriquez, 1972);
hemifacial hyperplasia syndromes (Pollock *et al.*, 1985).

16.3 Fissured tongues

Mild to moderate fissuring of the tongue appears to be a normal variant in 5-10% of the population. When very marked it has been called 'lingua fissurata'. Although usually present to some degree in trisomy-21, it can occur in otherwise completely normal people of high intelligence. It has been reported in abnormal syndromes of chromosome-11 but its remarkable association with trisomy-21 suggests that development and enfolding of the dorsum of the tongue and filiform papillae may be carried by chromosome-21. We have seen unusual variations of arrowhead fissures in association with no detected chromosome abnormalities (Levic *et al.*, 1975).

16.4 Lobulation and fusion defects

These are more commonly seen in association with other congenital defects and with intellectual handicap. The median area of *Candida* is now thought to occur widely. It is sometimes seen in fusion changes in the posterior septum or when minor labulations occur. It may also, in elderly patients, be well defined by chronic candidiasis as mentioned in the introductory section. This suggests that a central area of candidiasis is not merely a developmental abnormality, otherwise one would expect to see these changes more frequently in young people. Minor degrees of bifid changes towards the tip of the tongue are almost always associated with minor fusion defects in the midline or facial structures, or in association with intellectual handicap.

16.5 Ankyloglossia (or 'tongue-tie')

Abnormal development of the frenum of the tongue can occur to some minor degree in a wide range of normal children of different races. Sometimes the ankyloglossia (or 'tongue-tie') leads to later-than-normal speech development (Fernando & Glasson, 1983; Williams & Waldron, 1985). It is reported to be more common in Turner's and Klinefelter's syndromes but no statistical

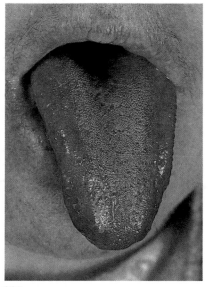 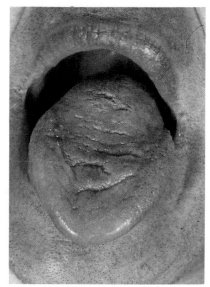

335 **336**

335 Treacher-Collins syndrome in a young woman with poor mandibular development, small tongue and no speech.

336 Microglossia with transverse fissures and some glossitis in an intellectually impaired microcephalic young man.

evidence for this could be found. 'Tongue-tie' is reported to be present in the oral-facial-digital syndrome. An abnormally long frenum can occur alone or in association with such disorders as Ehlers-Danlos syndrome. There is reported to be a danger in such children of tongue-swallowing, especially if the condition is associated with some intellectual impairment.

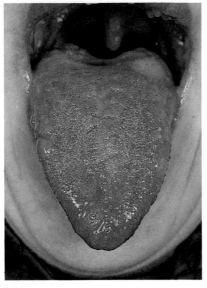 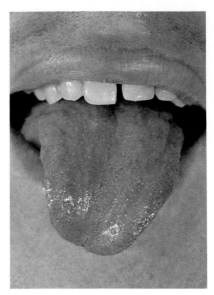

337   338

337 Relative microglossia with congenitally very large head and slow speech development. Some glossitis secondary to multiple anti-epileptic drugs.

338 Abnormal tongue tip (bifid tendency) since birth in 25-year-old unmarried man with intellectual impairment. No chromosome abnormality detected.

339 Congenital abnormality of the tongue with narrowing towards the tip and transverse fissures. Some mild glossitis.

340 Unusually large tongue in a microcephalic negro man. Probably due to growth of the tongue as a result of never wearing dentures.

341 Large fissured tongue in a 45-year-old man with Down's syndrome (trisomy-21).

342 Large, lobulated tongue in a markedly retarded 26-year-old man with no recognisable chromosomal abnormalities but many other multiple congenital defects.

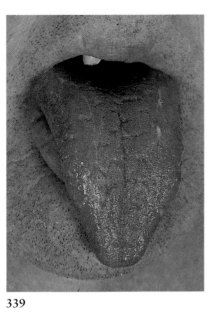

339

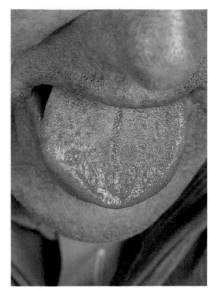

340

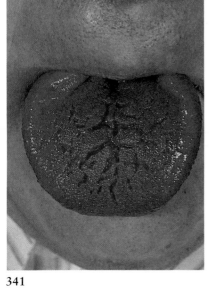

341

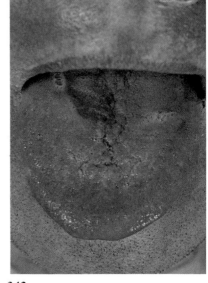

342

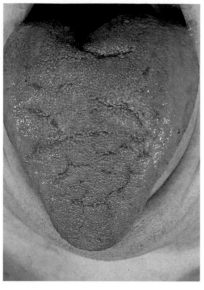
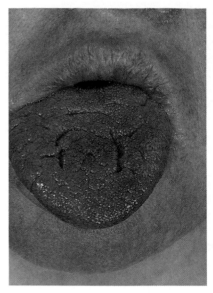

343   344

343 Tongue from 26-year-old man with Down's syndrome showing elongation, often described in this disorder, as well as an unusual fold posteriorly.

344 Fissures in tongue and also unusual fissures on the lips of a 36-year-old Down's syndrome patient.

345 Prematurely aged 30-year-old woman with trisomy-46. Short arm abnormality. With deletion on B4.

346 Marked transverse fissures in 54-year-old male diabetic otherwise normal. Congenital fissures since birth.

347 A 26-year-old male with Down's syndrome with small, irregular transverse fissures throughout a clean tongue.

348 Well-marked lateral fissures on both sides of the tongue in a 19-year-old male. Also deep mid-line fissure of unknown cause. No known pathology.

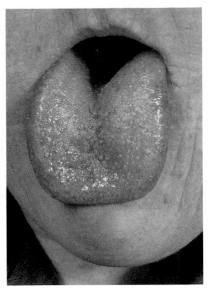

345

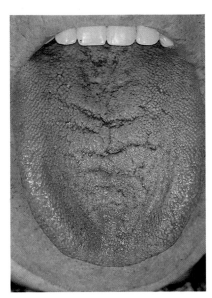

346

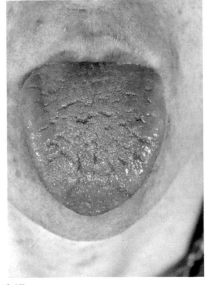

347

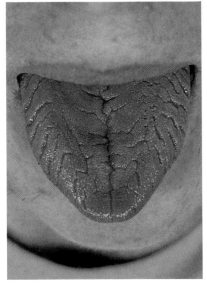

348

209

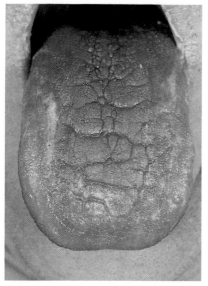

349

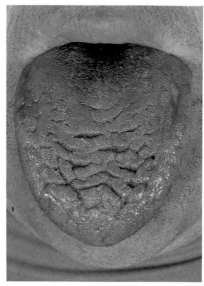

350

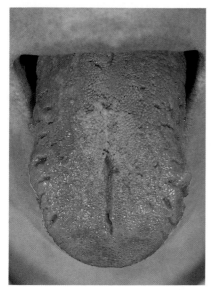

351

349 Large tongue from a Down's syndrome patient with glossitis and marked, widened fissures.

350 Deep transverse fissures in a 36-year-old Down's syndrome woman.

351 A deep longitudinal fissure, said to have been present since birth, in normal 36-year-old staff nurse.

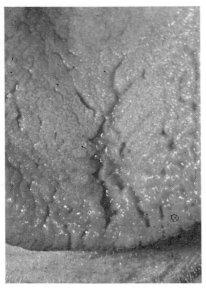

352

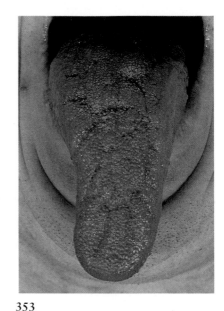

353

352 Unusual deep longitudinal fissure developing in elderly male with some glossitis. Unknown cause.

353 Elongated tongue in a Down's syndrome patient with 'crazy paving' fissures in the mid-tongue area.

354 Retarded 43-year-old male with suggestion of bifid tongue at the tip due to a very minor degree of congenital malunion.

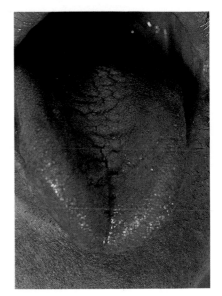

354

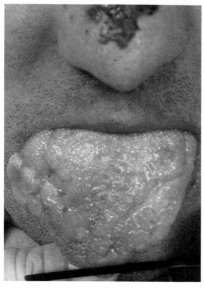 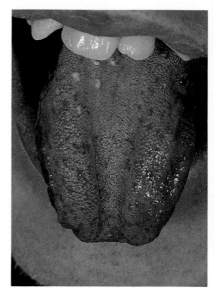

355   356

355   Unusual arrow markings in a tongue from a 'mosaic Down's syndrome' young man.

356   Some 'bifidness' of the tip of the tongue with some glossitis of edges present since birth in a 31-year-old woman. Note absence of lateral incisors.

357   Lobulated tongue since birth in 65-year-old dwarfed woman. Also marked lateral atrophy and general candidiasis.

358   A 29-year-old man with lobulated tongue cleaned from very obviously excessive mouth movements.

359   Large tongue from a trisomy-21 woman. Widespread small lobulations seen.

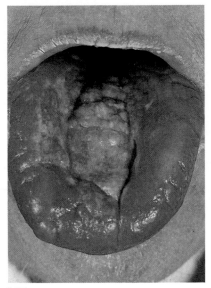

357

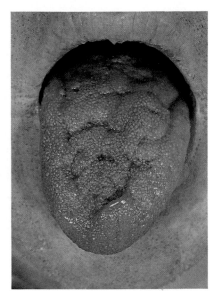

358

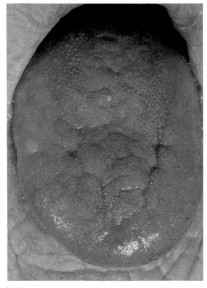

359

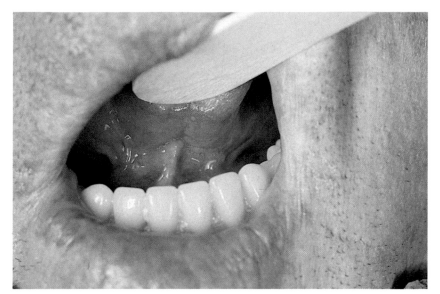

360

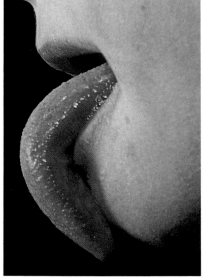

361

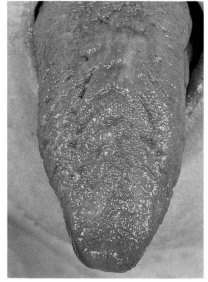

362

360 Congenitally short frenum with unusual fissures in 56-year-old man from isolated country area who had never learned to speak.

361 Congentially long frenum with very lax tongue in young teenage girl. No disabilities.

362 Another long tongue due to a lax frenum, this time with some early glossitis and mental impairment.

363 A 30-year-old male showing virtually absent frenum and a very lax tongue.

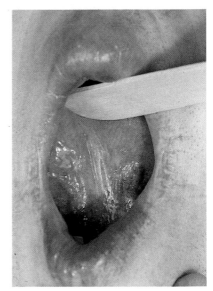

363

References

Boraz R.A., Hiebert J.M., Thomas M. Congenital micrognathia and microglossia: An experimental approach to treatment. *ASDC J Dentistry in Childhood* 1985, **52**(1), 62-64.

Fernando C., Glasson M.J. Speech therapy and surgery for tongue-tie: Abstract. *Aust Paediatr J* 1983, **19**(2), 119.

Grunt J.A., Enriquez A.R. Further studies of hypoglycemia in children with the examphalos-macroglossia-gigantism syndrome. *Yale J Biol & Med* 1972, **45**, 15-21.

Levic Z.M., Stefanovic B.S., Nikolic M.Z. *et al.* Progressive nuclear ophthalmoplegia associated with mental deficiency, lingua scrotalis and other neurological and ophthalmologic signs in a family. *Neurology* 1975, **25**, 68-71.

Pollock R.A., Newman M.H., Burdi A.R. *el al.* Congenital hemifacial hyperplasia: An embryologic hypothesis and case report. *Cleft Palate J* 1985, **22**(3), 173-184.

Williams W.N., Waldron C.M. Assessment of lingual function when ankyloglossia (tongue-tie) is suspected. *J Amer Dental Assn* 1985, **110**(3), 353-356.

Chapter 17
Palsies, Paralysis, Myoclonus and Muscle Disorders

The motor nerve to the tongue is the 12th cranial or hypoglossal nerve. This nerve is most commonly involved by damage or disease in its connections between the motor cortex and the nerve nucleus in the brain stem, thus giving an upper motor neurone lesion. Sites of pathological damage to the upper motor neurone above the nucleus are frequently in the internal capsule where the pyramidal tract fibres from the motor cortex collect together to enter the cerebro-spinal motor pathways. Involvement of the facial and tongue fibres of these pathways, either in the cortical regions or in the pyramidal tracts above the nucleus, will give some weakness on the affected site, so that the normal, stronger muscles on the unaffected side protrude the tongue outwards and round towards the affected side.

More commonly in ageing western-style populations, atheroma becomes increasingly common in the main-stem arteries to the brain. Thus these arteries and their branches which often turn off at sharp right angles, with subsequent haemodynamic disadvantage are much at risk. This has also increased because of the relative rapid growth over the last 2 million years of the brain. The changing flows and pressures of the upright posture worsen the haemodynamics. The lenticulo-striate branches of the middle cerebral arteries are frequently involved bilaterally. Repeated minor transient platelet emboli from the aortic arch or carotids adhere to the plaques forming at right angles in this area of blood vessels supplying the internal capsules on both sides of the brain.

Thus, repeated small lesions, often almost symptom-free, to the pyramidal tracts result in both sides of the tongue being gradually involved with increasing tone and slowness. Because of this slow course, over months or usually years, the tongue becomes spastic and wasted. No fasiculation or 'twitching' of the tongue takes place under such circumstances as there are bilateral upper motor neurone lesions, but 'snout' reflexes and the 'jaw jerk' should always be present.

Another important but rare cause of bilateral wasting is motor neurone disease. Here, slow loss of the 12th nerve nuclei due to an unknown cause leads to bilateral wasting of the tongue muscles with fasiculation in elderly patients. Fasiculation is best seen with the tongue at rest inside the mouth. It is exceptionally rare for both the motor nerves to the tongue to be otherwise involved.

In some reported cases of carcinoma of the floor of the mouth, there may be ipsilateral wasting and fasiculation. Otherwise, one of the 12th nerves may be involved by sub-mandibular hyperplasia, often called the Goldenhau syndrome (Miyamoto *et al.*, 1976) or due to a tumour of this secretory gland.

Any disorder or acute neuritis involving the course of the cranial nerves may also involve the hypoglossal or 12th nerve, as in some examples shown.

Apart from the more common wasting secondary to arterial disease in the elderly, and the very rare motor neurone disease in adult life, wasting of the tongue is unusual and difficult to detect (Dion *et al.*, 1984). Gross malnutrition and general wasting diseases from multiple secondary deposits may also involve the tongue, but even here it is often relatively spared.

In infancy or childhood, more severely affected family members with myotonia congenita or muscular dystrophies usually have functional disability and speech defects before wasting of the tongue is seen (Wyngaarden & Smith, 1982). Indeed, in lipid storage, myopathic syndromes such as the rarer triglyceride muscle disease or systemic or muscle carnitine deficiency states, the tongue remains at its normal size. In myasthenia gravis, eye signs and swallowing difficulties usually occur before chewing of food becomes a problem, and the tongue is not wasted, although some patients do complain of tongue tiredness. In tardive dyskinesis the tongue may show the so-called 'fly-catching' movements, but in its gross appearance it remains normal. Generalised myoclonic states, chorea and familial and acquired tremors can affect the tongue as they do other parts of the body. The outstretched tongue being a neuromuscular unit under functional pressure is a good site for detecting withdrawal tremors secondary to many drugs or alcohol. The degree of loss of force and mobility of the tongue in normal adults without neurological disease is still a matter of individual patient assessment and theoretical argument (Price & Darvell, 1981; Sonies *et al.*, 1984).

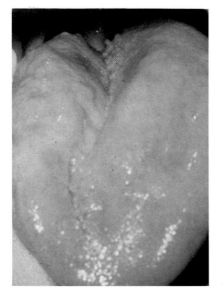

364

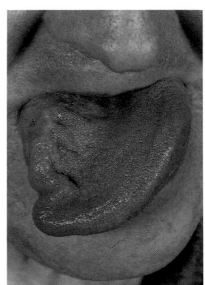

365

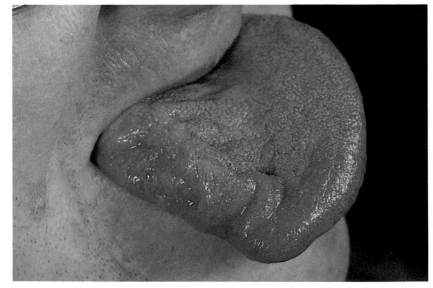

366

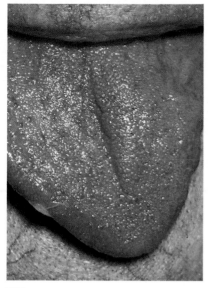

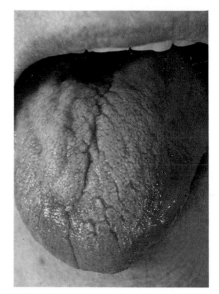

367   368

364   Recent left (L) lower motor neurone lesion of 12th cranial nerve in a 65-year-old woman with fibrosing submandibular disease.

365   Long-standing wasting of right hemi-tongue with tip protruded to the affected side after total excision of the 12th nerve several years previously.

366   Right lateral view of same tongue (365).

367   Partial weakness and wasting of left side of the tongue secondary to involvement of 3rd, 8th and 12th cranial nerves on the left side from marked Paget's disease of the skull.

368   Hemiatrophy (partial) due to hypoglossal nerve involvement from carcinoma of the sub-mandibular gland.

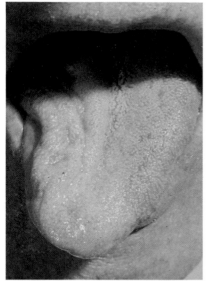

369

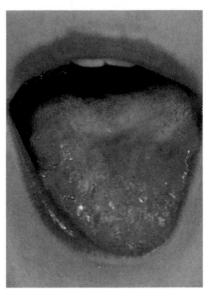

370

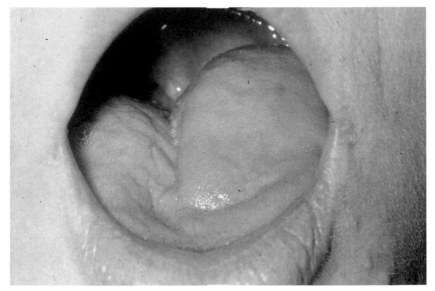

371

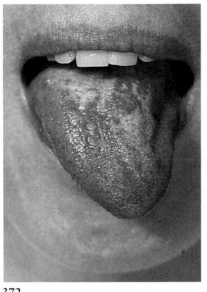
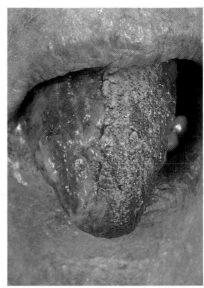

372   373

369   A 61-year-old man with marked wasting of the tongue and deviation due to a hypoglossal (12th) nerver tumour in the carotid body.

370   A minor degree of right 12th nerve palsy due to glomus tumour on the carotid body.

371   Partial recovery of right tongue hemiatrophy after hypoglossal facial nerve anastomosis.

372   Recent weakness and wasting of the tongue secondary to left lower 12th nerve palsy involved in cranial polyneuritis in a young housewife.

373   Herpes zoster infection involving the 12th nerve and right side of the tongue. A little wasting but no deviation.

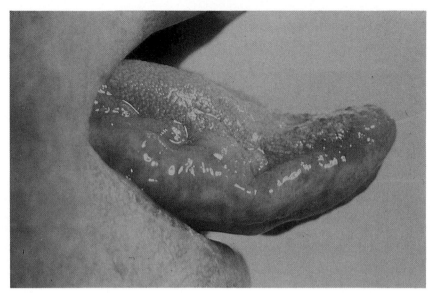

374

374 Wasting and weakness of the right half of the tongue seen from the right (R) side in a retired lawyer after post-carotid endarterectomy.

375 Hemiatrophy of the tongue and deviation to the left after cerebrovascular accident in the right internal capsule of the brain.

376 Left upper motor neurone damage involving the left side of the face and minimal deviation of the tongue to the left side.

377 Elderly man with left-sided stroke three months previously and almost complete recovery of tongue muscle power. Left tongue thinner and less coated.

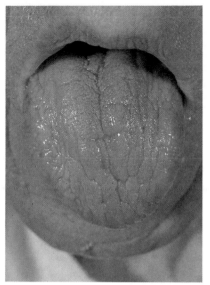

375

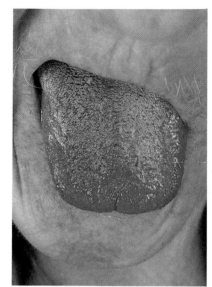

376

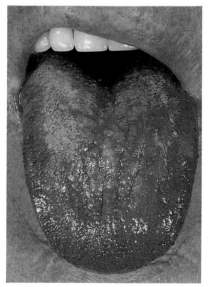

377

223

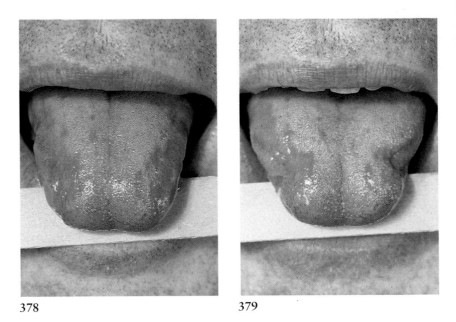

378

379

378 and 379   Myoclonus of the tongue showing normal tongue resting on a throat stick. After percussion, the tongue continues to contract on both sides.

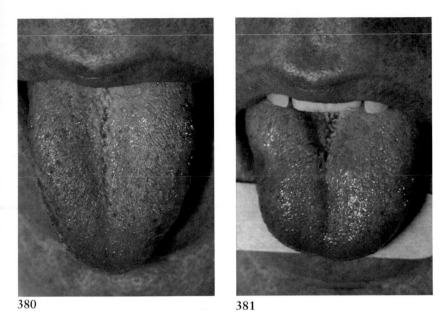

380   381

380 and 381   Myotonia of the tongue in a brother of previous patient (378 and 379) showing normal tongue and contracture of the muscles after tapping.

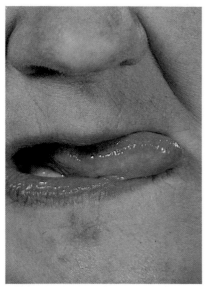

382

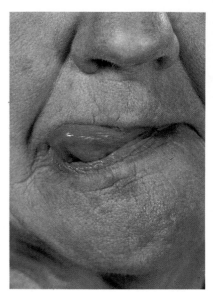

383

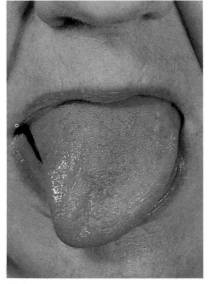

384

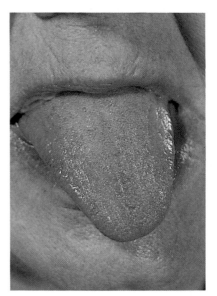

385

382-385 Rapid movements of the tongue photographed at half-second intervals in an elderly woman with severe drug-induced tardive dyskinesis.

References

Dion J.E., Fox A.J., Pelz D. *et al.* CT demonstration of hemiatrophy and fatty replacement of the tongue. *J Can Assn Rad* 1984, 35(4), 395-396.

Miyamoto R.T., Hamaker R.C., Lingeman R.E. Goldenhau syndrome associated with submandibular gland hyperplasia and hemihypoplasia of the mobile tongue. *Arch Otolaryngol* 1976, **102**, 313-314.

Price P.A., Darvell B.W. Force and mobility in the ageing human tongue. *Med J Aust* 1981, **1**, (2), 75-8.

Sonies B.C., Baum B.J., Shawker T.H. Tongue motion in elderly adults: Initial *in situ* observations. *J Gerontol* 1984, 39(3), 279-283.

Wyngaarden J.B., Smith L.H. *Cecil's Textbook of Medicine,* 16th edn. W.B. Saunders, New York, 1982.

Chapter 18

Tumours, Haemangiomas, Cysts, Ranulas and Cancers

Because of the great vascularity of the tongue, *haemangiomata* are common. Although sometimes described as 'cavernous' or 'capillary' on histological grounds, it is now believed that these are mostly of developmental origin, arising from primitive vascular tissue. Smaller haemangiomata, particularly of the multiple inherited type such *as hereditary haemorrhagic telangiectasia* (Osler-Rendu-Weber disease) may present because of their bleeding tendency. These blobs, spots or spider-like angiomata are also almost always seen on the buccal surface of the lips as well as on the tongue. Their importance and those of the other rarer angiomata is that they occur in other sites of the embryonic foregut and therefore lead to upper gastro-intestinal bleeding from the oesophagus or stomach. In such disorders, the abnormal blood vessels on the surface are surrounded by abnormal elastic tissue which later stretches to permit dilatation and bleeding.

Other haemangiomata (and rarely, haematomas) can initially be small or sessile or, with growth, can become pedunculated. Major haemangiomata tend to have a soft surface and easily undergo minor trauma with bleeding. When associated with connective tissue, as in sclerosing haemangiomata, the lesions may be pale pink and much firmer to palpation. Larger, deeply seated haemangiomata in the tongue can give quite marked macroglossia. Diagnosis is confirmed by bilateral palpation (as described in methods of examining the tongue in Chapter 2) and confirmed by local angiography or ultrasound.

Other simple tumours may occur in the tongue such as salivary neoplasms. Others even more rare can usually only be accurately diagnosed by specialist referral (Weisenfeld *et al.*, 1983) and early biopsy to make the diagnosis of *fibrosis* (Laskaris *et al.*, 1981), *xanthomas* or granulomas (Sklavounou *et al.*, 1982; Elzay, 1983) or *rare developmental tumours* (Gardner & Corio, 1983; Reychler *et al.*, 1983). *Benign lingual lesions* deserve a careful differential diagnosis (Newland, 1984)) and may only be *slowly growing chondromas* (Segal *et al.*, 1984) or *ectopic osteomata*.

Any suggestion of *tongue cancer*, whether starting from symptoms of persistent ulceration, a fullness in the base or root of the tongue or white areas with hypertrophic or dysphasic changes (Ortiz *et al.*, 1982) demands the following.

A decision on whether there is some abnormality present which means mandatory referral to a specialist. Oral medicine specialists will see many referred cases even in minority groups (Merchant *et al.*, 1986).

A specialist opinion on biopsy and cytology following an accurate bimanual examination of the tongue in a good light is required.

This whole topic of tongue cancer is a complex, large and specialised one which cannot be covered in a small visual guide. However, recent emphasis in the literature has been on early diagnosis (McDaniel, 1984; Newman *et al.*, 1983) and a readiness to biopsy areas of leukoplakia. Subsequently, the decision to biopsy suspected lesions on the surface or deeper in the tongue tissue can be made with or without help (particularly in difficult large or deep lesions) by CT scan, ultrasound or angiography. Other lesions of the tongue such as myomas, myoblastomas, cysts and ranulas, will all need expert help in diagnosis. Risk factors for tongue cancer (Chen, 1981; Vermund *et al.*, 1982) appear to be:

male;
age 45 to 80 years (maximum rates);
smoking;
high alcohol intake;
multiple-malignancy families;
poor oral hygiene;
betel chewing habit;
malnutrition.

In critical reviews, colour and race are not supported as factors (McCarthy & Shklar, 1980). Some observers classify by gross histology, such as papillary or verrucous, ulcerative, infiltrative, scirrhous, but the international classification developed in 1967, although modified, remains the basis for staging procedures.

Plummer-Vinson or Paterson-Kelly syndrome (atrophy of tongue, post-cricoid web with oesophageal and gastric mucous membrane with iron deficiency anaemia and koilonychia), and avitaminosis B in animal studies, although rarer, seem to be accepted as risk factors in the development of cancer of the oral cavity.

Carcinomas are by far the commonest form of malignancy of the tongue.

Sarcomas and pseudosarcomas (Ferrando *et al.*, 1983) may sometimes present to the oral medicine specialist with this diagnosis. Treatment programmes of deeper and invasive cancers remain challenging and highly specialised. (Yamamoto *et al.*, 1983; Thawley *et al.*, 1983; Wadler *et al.*, 1985.)

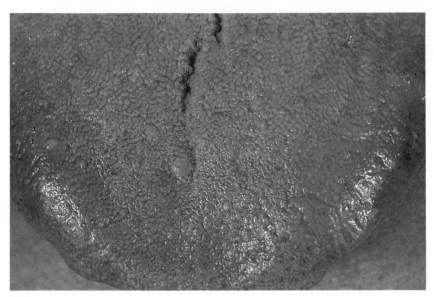

386

386 Small papilloma near the central fissure towards the tip of the tongue in a 53-year-old chain-smoker of cigars.

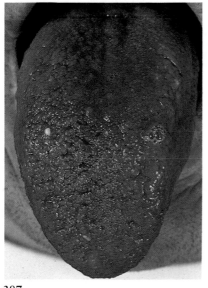
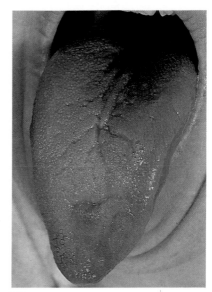

387

388

387 A very small papilloma on the posterior central tongue amongst hypertrophied vallate papillae.

388 A non-malignant papilloma in an elderly woman with some cheilitis.

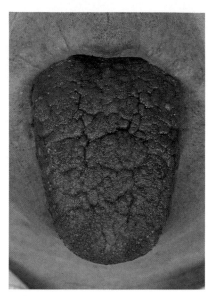

389

389 Several micro-papillomata arising in hypertrophied areas in an older tongue with very long history of chronic hypertrophic glossitis.

390 Fibro-epithelial polyps.

391 'Fungating' papilloma of the tongue.

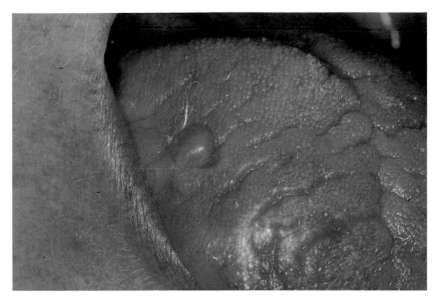

390

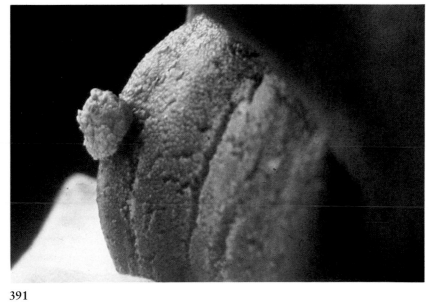

391

233

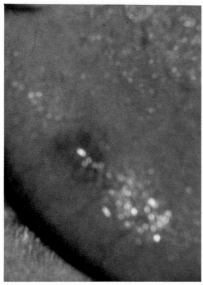

392

392 A small haemangioma in the right border of the tongue of a Maori man.

393 Large fungating haemangioma in a young woman referred for surgery.

394 Long sessile haemangioma in the left border of the tongue posteriorly.

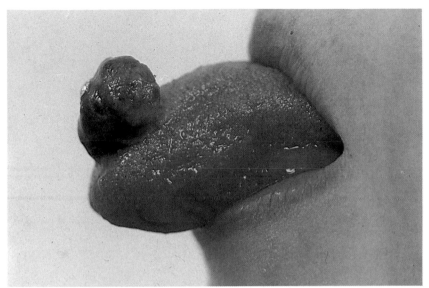

393

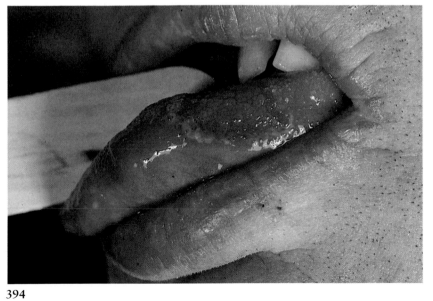

394

235

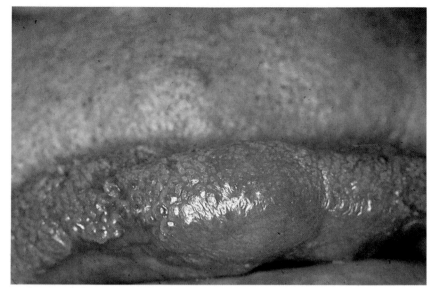

395

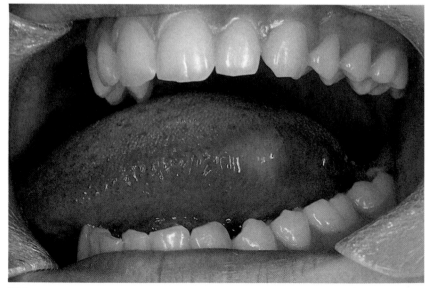

396

236

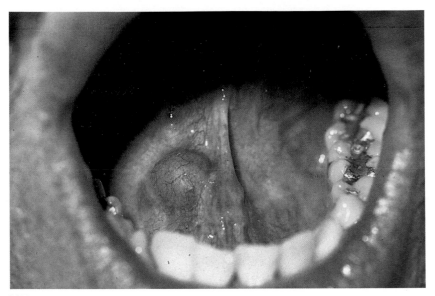

397

395 Lipoma at the tip of the tongue in an elderly man.

396 Small fibroma on the left side near the tip of the tongue in a teenager.

397 Typical ranula or retention cyst on the floor of the mouth (*ranula* = 'frog-like skin').

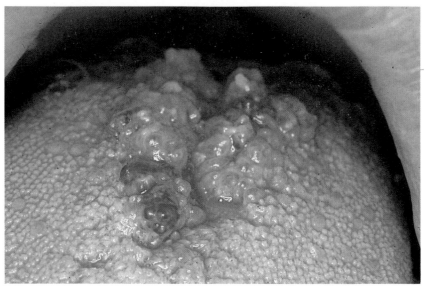

398

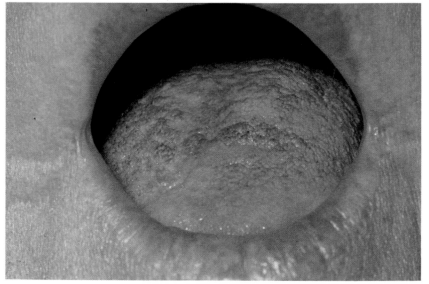

399

238

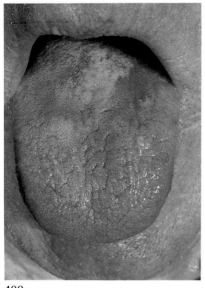
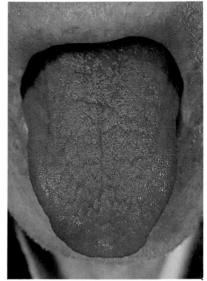

400   401

398 Lymphosarcoma arising in posterior third of the lymphoid structures of the tongue.

399 Carcinoma *in situ* on the dorsum of the tongue.

400 Very small carcinoma *in situ* arising in atrophied area on the left edge posteriorly. Minor long-standing geographic tongue.

401 Rapidly growing vascular tumour near the tip on the right side of the tongue in a heavy-smoking male. Probably cancerous, referred for biopsy.

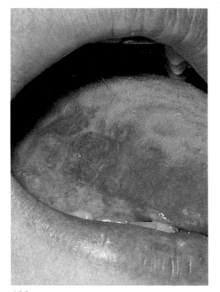

402

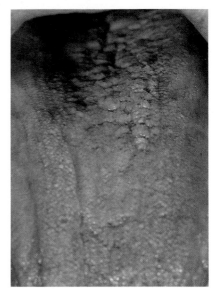

403

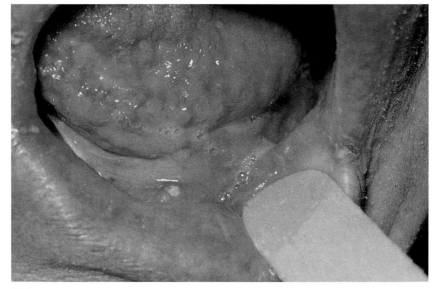

404

240

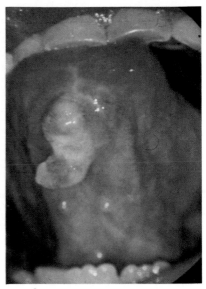

405

402 Carcinoma *in situ* in a 20-year-old woman arising in lichenoid area.

403 Malignant melanoma in a 73-year-old woman. The lesion is in the right posterior tongue in an area of leukoplakia.

404 Sessile or verrucous carcinoma along the floor of the mouth on the left side of the tongue.

405 Small papillary cancer on the ventral surface of the tongue.

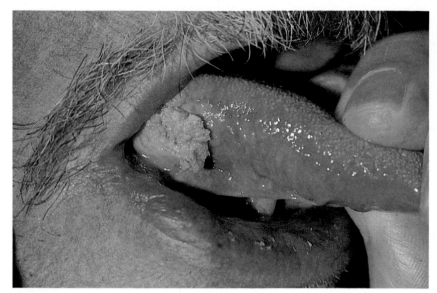

406

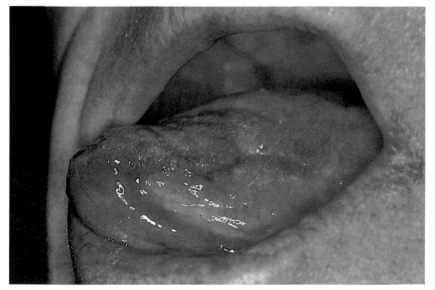

407

242

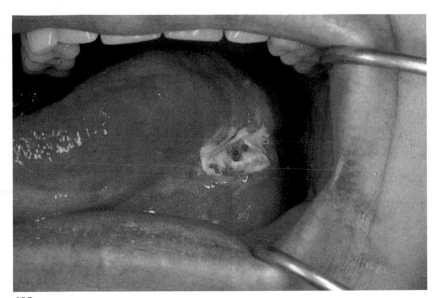

408

406 Large papillary cancer under posterior third of the lateral edge in a 59-year-old heavy pipe-smoking man.

407 Erosive cancer near the tip of the tongue. Note also angular stomatitis.

408 Small squamous cell cancer in an elderly woman posteriorly.

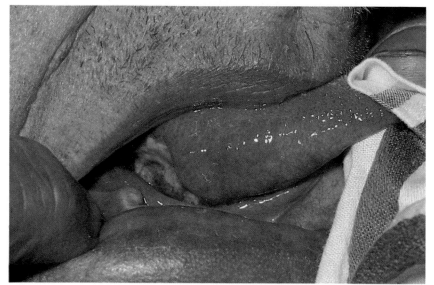

409

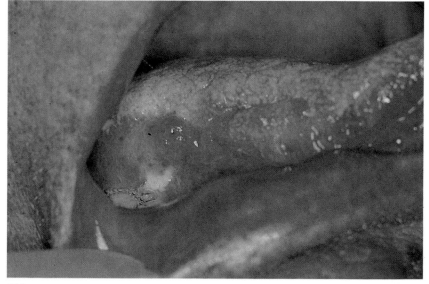

410

244

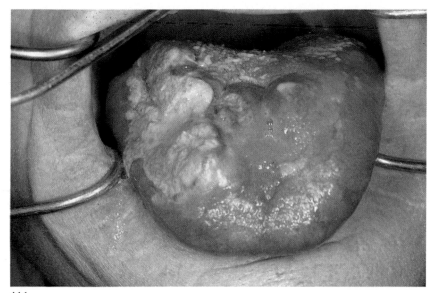

411

409 Large sloughing ulcer in posterior ventral tongue. Infiltrative carcinoma.

410 Peduncular tumour in the posterior lateral tongue in a 57-year-old farmer – ulcerating below.

411 Scirrhous carcinoma in the posterior third of the tongue on the right.

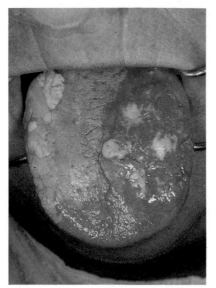

412

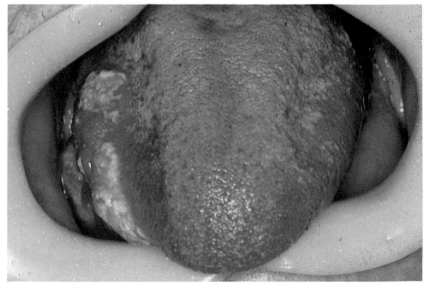

413

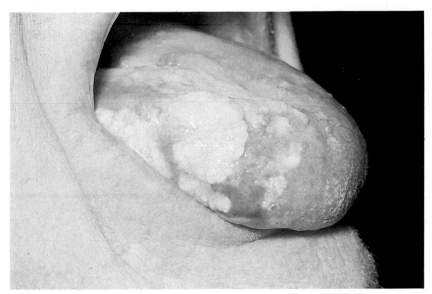

414

412 Extensive squamous cell carcinoma in a 79-year-old woman. Note also the patch of leukoplakia on the right border of the tongue posteriorly.

413 Verrucous cancer extensively infiltrating the base of a black hairy tongue on the right side.

414 Carcinoma *in situ* arising in the front edge of an extensive area of leukoplakia.

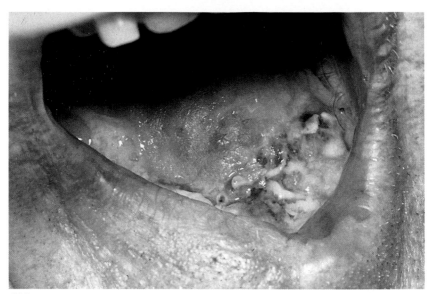

415

415 Extensive recurrent carcinoma in the floor of the mouth with scirrhous tongue from previous radiation treatment.

References

Chen Z.L. Investigation on tongue appearances of 1046 patients with malignant tumor compared with those of 500 healthy subjects as controls. *Chung Hsi I Chieh Ho Tsa Chih* 1981, **1**(2), 81-83.

Elzay R.P. Traumatic ulcerative granuloma with stromal eosinophilia (Riga-Fede's disease) and traumatic eosinophilic granuloma. *Oral Surg Oral Med Oral Path* 1983, **55**(5), 497-506.

Ferrando J., Palou J., Mascaro J.M. *et al*. Polypoid pseudosarcoma of the tongue. *Med Cutan Iber Lat Am* 1983, **11**(5), 343-348.

Gardner D.G., Corio R.L. Fetal rhabdomyoma of the tongue with a discussion of the two histologic variants of this tumor. *Oral Surg Oral Med Oral Path* 1983, **56**(3), 293-300.

Inoue A., Sakamoto A., Tsuzuku M. *et al*. Early invasive squamous cell carcinoma of the tongue. Report of a case. *Gan No Rinsho* 1985, **31**(1), 83-86.

Laskaris G., Bovopoulou O., Nicolis G. Oral submucous fibrosis in a Greek female. *Br J Oral Surg* 1981, **19**(3), 197-201.

McCarthy P.I.., Shklar G. *Epidemiology of Oral Cancer and Aetiologic factors.* 2nd edn. Lea & Febiger, Philadelphia, 1980, pp479-492.

McDaniel P.K. Lingual malignancies. Improving early detection and diagnosis. *Postgrad Med* 1984, 75(4), 173-185.

Merchant N.E., Ferguson M.M. *et al.*, Oral carcinoma in the Indian and Pakistani population in Scotland. *J Oral Med* 1986, **41**, 62-65.

Newland J.R. Benign lingual lesions of intrinsic origin. Differential diagnosis. *Postgrad Med* 1984, 75(4), 151-163.

Newman A.N., Rice D.H., Ossoff R.H. *et al.* Carcinoma of the tongue in persons younger than 30 years of age. *Arch Otolaryngol* 1983, **109**(5), 302-304.

Ortiz M.J., Fay J.T., Weir G.T. Heterotopic gastric mucosa of the tongue. *J Oral Maxillofac Surg* 1982, 40(10), 667-670.

Segal K., Sidi J., Katzav Y., *et al.* Chondroma of the tongue. Report of two cases. *Ann Otol Rhinol Laryngol* 1984, 93(3), 271-272.

Sklavounou A., Laskaris G., Angelopoulos A. Verruciform xanthoma of the oral mucosa. *Dermatologica* 1982, **164**(1), 41-46.

Thawley S.E., Simpson J.R., Marks J.E. *et al.* Pre-operative irradiation and surgery for carcinoma of the base of the tongue. *Ann Otol Rhinol Laryngol* 1983, **92**(5 Part 1), 485-490.

Vermund H., Brennhovid I.O., Kaalhus O. *et al.* Carcinoma of the tongue in Norway and Wisconsin. II. Influence of site and clinical stage on local control of the tumor. *Acta Radio (Oncol)* 1982, **21**(4), 209-216.

Wadler S., Muller R., Spigelman M.K. *et al.* Fulminant disseminated carcinomatosis arising from squamous cell carcinoma of the tongue. *Amer J Med* 1985, **78**(1), 149-152.

Weisenfeld D., Ferguson M.M., McMillan N. Simultaneous computed tomography and sialography of the parotid and submandibular glands. *Brit J Oral Surg* 1983, **21**, 268.

Yamamoto E., Sunakawa H., Kohama G. Clincial course of diffuse invasive carcinoma of the tongue excised after bleomycin treatment. *J Maxillofac Surg* 1983, **11**(6), 269-274.

Chapter 19
Specialised Examinations

Once an abnormal lesion has been identified, the patient needs to be referred to a specialist in oral medicine or surgery who is fully conversant with the indications for all investigations. It is not within the scope of this small visual guide to mainly *common* appearances of the tongue, to discuss the virtues of different ancillary aids to diagnosis. Early and adequate biopsy with interpretation and collaboration by an experienced and well-trained colleague in histopathology is clearly essential. All clinicians or health workers who have a responsibility to look into the mouth need to be aware that this *is* a neglected clinical area. Curiosity is the hallmark of the excellent clinical observer (Richards, 1986). Well-staffed departments of oral medicine and surgery should have ready access to the following.

Biopsy and standard histopathology (Morgan *et al.*, 1984).
Specialised histochemical and fluorescence-activated antibody staining techniques (Thompson, 1984; Dhillon & Rode, 1983; Hartzband *et al.*, 1984).
Electron microscopy (Dourov, 1984) of biopsied material.
Pertechnate scans can be used to identify small lumps which can be shown to be aberrant 'lingual' thyroid tissue.
Ultrasound examination of the tongue (Miller, 1985; Morrish *et al.*, 1984).
Computerised tomography of the body and base of the tongue.
Positron emission tomography and magnetic resonance imaging (MRI).
This very expensive equipment gives more definition of small lesions in solid inaccessible areas such as the body and root of the tongue.

References

Dhillon A.P., Rode J. Immunohistochemical studies of S100 protein and other neural characteristics expressed by granular cell tumor. *Diagn Histopathol* 1983, 6(1), 23-28.

Dourrov N. Scanning electron microscopy contribution in oral pathology. *Scan Electron Microsc* 1984, (1), 243-248.

Hartzband P.I., Diehl D.L., Lewin K.J. *et al.* Histological characterisation of a lingual mass using thyroglobulin immunoperoxidase staining. *J Endocrinol Invest* 1984, 7(3), 221-3.

Miller J.H. Lingual thyroid gland. Sonographic appearance. *Radiology* 1985, 156(1), 83-84.

Morgan R.F., Friedman H.I., Johns M.E. Use of the Satinsky clamp for excision of anterior tongue lesions. *Amer Surg* 1984, 50(12), 677-678.

Morrish K.A., Stone M., Sonies B.C. *et al.* Characterisation of tongue shape. *Ultrasonic Imaging* 1984, 6(1), 37-47.

Richards P. Clinical competence and curiosity. *Br Med J* 1986, 292, 1481-1482.

Thompson S.H. Myoglobin content of granular cell tumour of the tongue. An immunoperoxidase study. *Oral Surg Oral Med Oral Path* 1984, 57(1), 74-76.

Index